PRE-OBJECT RELATEDNESS

The Guilford Psychoanalysis Series

Robert S. Wallerstein, Editor

Associate Editors

Leonard Shengold
Neil J. Smelser
Albert J. Solnit
Edward M. Weinshel

PRE-OBJECT RELATEDNESS
Early Attachment and the Psychoanalytic Situation
  Ivri Kumin

THE PROBLEM OF TRUTH IN APPLIED
PSYCHOANALYSIS
  Charles Hanly

HALO IN THE SKY
Observations on Anality and Defense
  Leonard Shengold

FROM SAFETY TO SUPEREGO
Selected Papers of Joseph Sandler
  Joseph Sandler

THE TEACHING AND LEARNING
OF PSYCHOANALYSIS
Selected Papers of Joan Fleming, M.D.
  Stanley S. Weiss, Editor

FORTY-TWO LIVES IN TREATMENT
A Study of Psychoanalysis and Psychotherapy
  Robert S. Wallerstein

PRE-OBJECT RELATEDNESS

Early Attachment and the Psychoanalytic Situation

Ivri Kumin, M.D.

THE GUILFORD PRESS
New York   London

© 1996 The Guilford Press
A Division of Guilford Publications, Inc.
72 Spring Street, New York, NY 10012

Printed in the United States of America

This book is printed on acid-free paper.

Last digit is print number: 9 8 7 6 5 4 3 2 1

Library of Congress Cataloging-in-Publication Data

Kumin, Ivri.
    Pre-object relatedness: early attachment and the psychoanalytic
situation / Ivri Kumin.
        p.   cm.—(The Guilford Psychoanalysis series)
    Includes bibliographical references and index.
    ISBN 1-57230-015-9
    1. Object relations (Psychoanalysis) 2. Attachment behavior.
  3. Emotions in infants. 4. Ego (Psychology). 5. Psychoanalysis.
I. Title. II. Series.
BF175.5.O24K85 1996
155.42′28—dc20   95-19657
                                                                    CIP

For Linda, Avi, and Esther
and for my mother and father

Shapeless and impalpable ourselves, we want
that reality which has no shape to occupy.

—WILLIAM BRONK
Vectors and Smoothable Curves

. . . the patient must go on looking for the past
detail which is *not yet experienced.*

—D. W. WINNICOTT
Fear of Breakdown

Acknowledgments

ONE OF THE EARLIEST influences on the writing of this book was a brief letter I received in 1976 from Clare Winnicott. I had written to her to tell her how much I appreciated the work of her late husband. She wrote back and included a paper, "Fear of Breakdown," published after Winnicott's death. In it Winnicott traced the adult fear of a future mental breakdown to a fear of a breakdown that has *already* occurred—but that occurred so early in life it cannot be remembered. Winnicott poignantly described how the past breakdown must reoccur in the transference, as though for the first time, in order to be fully encompassed. It is only now, after completing this book, that I realize just how much I was influenced by Clare Winnicott's letter and by the reprint she enclosed.

I am grateful to several mentors. Arthur Epstein of the Tulane Psychoanalytic Medicine Program, a teacher of mine in medical school, was the first person to encourage me to become an analyst. When I entered training, Art supervised my first cases, urged me to publish, and provided me opportunities to teach and eventually to codirect the training program with him. Don Rinsley of Topeka also fostered my early psychoanalytic development over years of always brilliant and often very funny correspondence. The idea of my writing a book originated with him shortly before his premature death. Henry Krystal wrote to me after coming across a paper of mine that he liked and has, ever since, treated me to his warmth, enthusiasm, and generosity. His experience, knowledge, and broad-based scholarship have been constant models for me. Charlie Mangham of the Seattle Institute for Psychoanalysis first opened my eyes to the relevance of infant development research to psychoanalytic practice.

He brought to my attention Meltzoff's research on intermodal matching at the University of Washington, read early chapters of this book, and encouraged me to continue at a point when I was feeling particularly discouraged about the slow progress I was making. My two training analysts, Lillian Robinson at Tulane and Ted Dorpat in Seattle, were also instrumental in my personal and psychoanalytic development.

Bob Wallerstein was the North American editor of the *International Review of Psycho-Analysis* who accepted my first two papers for publication in 1978. Ten years later he was the editor of a psychoanalytic book series for The Guilford Press and convinced Seymour Weingarten, Guilford's Editor-in-Chief, to accept my proposal for this book. I deeply appreciate the encouragement both of them gave me. Guilford's excellent editors made the production process pleasurable. Kitty Moore, the editor at Guilford who worked with me to publish the final version of the book, helped immeasurably with her warmth and support no less than with her keen understanding of psychoanalytic theory and practice. The copy editor, Toby Troffkin, often knew what I wanted to say better than I did myself, and the Senior Production Editor, Anna Brackett, worked closely with me during the process of turning my manuscript into a book.

I also am grateful to those clinicians who were willing to take time away from their work to read and comment on individual chapters of this book. They include George Allison, Katalina Bartok, Romalee Davis, Hugh Dickinson, Arthur Epstein, Edward Freedman, Henry Krystal, Ronald Levin, Michael Mandel, Stephen Maurer, Andrew Meltzoff, Gerald Olch, James Raney, Anne-Marie Sandler, Evelyne Schwaber, Robert Stolorow, Frances Tustin, and Vann Spruiell. I appreciate the help from members of the child psychoanalysis faculty study group of the Seattle Institute for Psychoanalysis, including Gene Bauman, Adolph Gruhn, Kenneth King, Linda McDonald, Charles Mangham, Gerald Olch, and Werner Schimmelbusch, who read and commented on portions of the book while I was completing final editing.

Some of the help I received came in casual and unexpected ways: Ed Freedman helped me refine some of my ideas about affect regulation while we drove together to a round of golf; Mike Mandel reminded me of Spitz's work on the pre-objectal phase and Steve Maurer introduced me to Kinston and Cohen's papers on primal repression during chats about committee work for the Seattle Institute for Psychoanalysis; over barbecue at a mutual friend's home, Rob Janes offered a valuable suggestion that helped me complete the book, and I discussed relevant ideas with Sue Betts, Bob Campbell, Jeanette Dyal, Frederick Hoedemaker, Ken King, Nick McConaughy, Nels Magelssen, and Roberta Myers between appointments in the hallway of our shared offices. A friend and neighbor, Wayne Morse, generously shared his extensive first-hand knowledge of the production side of medical publishing and offered practical suggestions that facilitated my completion of the book.

Various regional organizations nurtured and supported the book's progress by providing forums for me to present my developing ideas, including especially the Seattle Institute for Psychoanalysis, the Northwest Alliance for Psychoanalytic Study, the Vancouver, British Columbia, Psychoanalytic Psychotherapy Society, and the British Object Relations Group. I also want to thank the Tulane Division of Psychoanalytic Medicine in New Orleans, my first psychoanalytic school. Tulane's is the rare psychoanalytic training program that is integrated into a department of psychiatry. There, as a recent medical graduate, I was able to begin my psychoanalytic education concurrently with my psychiatric residency. I am convinced that the integration of psychoanalysis with university education is the best way to train psychoanalysts. Later I also completed a second training with the Seattle Institute for Psychoanalysis, where I was introduced to the developmental approach by its child psychoanalytic instructors.

Finally, I would like to thank my patients. Trusting in me, they relived often painful early experiences. I hope I have understood enough of what they needed me to understand.

Contents

III. PATHOLOGY OF PRE-OBJECT RELATEDNESS

PRE-OBJECT RELATEDNESS

Introduction

MUCH OF THE RECENT HISTORY of psychoanalytic research has focused on the study of the earliest dimensions of human experience. This is in part an effort to expand the frontier of psychoanalytic knowledge to developmentally earlier periods of mental and emotional development than that of the Oedipus complex and thus to periods of development that predate the formation of the tripartite structure of the mind. The interest in this endeavor is partly created by the nature of psychoanalytic work, which inevitably presents us with evidence of the extensiveness as well as the limitations of our understanding.

Our goal as psychoanalysts and researchers is in some ways paradoxical: to conduct our analyses so deeply that we reach at times to those realms of the personality that are preanalyzable. The current psychoanalytic interest in neonatal research and studies of attachment behavior is evidence of the fervent effort to encompass within psychoanalytic theory and practice a better understanding of infancy. Such knowledge not only assists us in expanding the scope of psychoanalytic treatment to the more developmentally disturbed patients who increasingly consult us for help but also enables us to be more searching in the analyses of even our best-integrated patients for the sources of disturbances that may have their origins in periods of development that predated the patient's capacity to represent self-experience in verbal terms. As analysts of Oedipal conflict we search for the child in our adult patients, but as analysts of pre-Oedipal disturbances we search for the infant in them. If we succeed in this search, if we help our patients to find these earliest experiences within themselves, we are presented with aspects of the transference that to some extent predate memory, predate symbolic representation and verbal description, predate self-reflection, and predate the conscious awareness of the contribution of the original caretaker and of the analyst. We approach the foundation of affect itself, and with this approach the patient's ability to regulate his or her own emotions often alters permanently for the better.

Psychoanalysis began as a study of the vicissitudes of drives and unconscious wishes. Freud never stopped trying to understand how these instinctual forces were tamed. Early in his career he conceptualized the process in terms of the damming up of drive tension and its subsequent release. As his theory matured, he introduced a personified theory of internal mental structures derived from a compromise between the imperatives of unconscious wishes and the realities of human relationships. Near the end of his life he admitted the limitations of what he had learned when he wrote the following:

> If we are asked by what methods and means this [taming of the instinct] is achieved, it is not easy to find an answer. We can only say: "So muss denn doch die Hexe dran!" ["We must call the Witch to our help after all!"—Goethe, *Faust*, Part 1, Scene 6]—the Witch Metapsychology. Without metapsychological speculation and theorizing—I had almost said "phantasying"—we shall not get another step forward. Unfortunately, here as elsewhere, what our Witch reveals is neither very clear nor very detailed. We have only a single clue to start from—though it is a clue of the highest value—namely, the antithesis between the primary and the secondary processes. (Freud, 1937, p. 225)

I suggest that the antithesis between primary and secondary processes referred to by Freud is derived from the internalized gradient between the primitive mental apparatus of the infant and the emotional mediation of its mother. In this sense Goethe's Witch, the magical woman who is summoned for help, is the omnipotent mother of our infancy. It is initially the infant's mother who, by holding and soothing it and by her ongoing attempt to understand the nature of its discomforts, tames (or fails to tame) the baby's instincts. Later, when the infant matures, it acquires the capacity to regulate its emotional states, as its mother once did, for itself. In other words, the drive-taming functions of the individual's ego are derived in part from an internalization of the infant–mother relationship.

Such an orientation inevitably requires a theory of preautonomous relational modes. Many psychoanalytic authors have tried to understand the nature of the emotional experience in infancy. The major contributions to this field began with Freud's studies of the presymbolic "body ego" of infancy. Soon afterward, Melanie Klein began to describe phases in the development of the infant's internal world and Wilfred Bion studied primitive pathology in the creation of thought. D. W. Winnicott contributed an understanding of the crucial role of good-enough environmental support in the establishment of psychosomatic integrity and continuity of being in infancy. René Spitz initiated his observations of foundling home infants. Esther Bick pioneered the field of psychoanalytic infant observation. John Bowlby began his ethological studies of infant attachment and loss, and Mary Ainsworth helped invent the "Strange Situation" experiment to follow its effects. Margaret Mahler studied the earliest experiences of the individuation process. Paul Federn, Bertram Lewin, and Heinz Hartmann explored the most primitive functioning of the ego. Edith Jacobson, Joseph Sandler, and Otto Kernberg described the early development of the representational world. Heinz Kohut focused on the experience of a cohesive sense of self, and Robert Stolorow described the fundamental intersubjectivity that subserves or derails the development of that cohesion. Henry Krystal investigated the wellsprings of affect and the effect of trauma. Frances Tustin and Thomas Ogden traced autistic deconstruction of human connection to its earliest developmental influences. Michel de M'Uzan, Didier Anzieu, and other French analysts linked psychosomatic disorders to disturbances of early ego functioning, and Graeme Taylor in Canada described psychosomatic disturbance in terms of the dysregulation of affects. Emde, Greenspan, Sander, Stern, and other contemporary researchers are pioneering a new science of infant developmental studies.

While all of these authors and their explicators have tended to emphasize the differences in their approaches and their views, and while these differences are indeed substantive, this book highlights their similarities, the areas of what Wallerstein (1990) describes as the "common ground" of psychoanalysis that are somehow undervalued. Despite their differences, many of these authors describe early ego experiences similarly. I refer to this earliest dimension of experience as "pre-object relatedness." Pre-object relatedness denotes a modality of experience that develops prior to the baby's conscious, reflective awareness of itself and others as being real, permanent, independently motivated individuals. Pre-object relatedness is characterized by the preverbal exchange of emotional shape and regulatory function between mother and infant and persists as a background capacity in all interpersonal communication throughout life. Pre-object relatedness is, in a sense, a generic term. Part-objects, selfobjects, transitional objects, bizarre objects, and anaclitic objects—all such developmentally primitive experiential configurations are types of pre-object experience.

Scientific progress is made when an understanding is reached that all of the elements that were previously thought to be disparate are actually parts of a whole that is more complex than any of its individual components. So, too, with our attempts to understand very early human development. Certainly, to the extent that we are attempting to describe preverbal realms of experience, words will always fail us. However, in bringing together these common elements between varieties of early experience, the chapters in this book relate loosely to Freud's unanswered question about the means by which the instincts are tamed—and to the "single clue" he left us.

PART ONE

The Basic Language
of Primary Relatedness

CHAPTER ONE

Attachment to the Unperceived

> I have long surmised that not only the repressed
> content of the psyche, but also the . . . core of our
> ego is unconscious. . . . I infer this from the fact
> that consciousness is . . . a sensory organ directed
> toward the outside world, so that it is always
> attached to a part of the ego which is itself
> unperceived."
>
> *—Sigmund Freud, in a letter to
> LudwigBinswanger (July 4, 1912)*[1]

ANY CONSIDERATION of the ego's core approximates an embryology of human relatedness. Thus, one might interpret Freud's statement above as an indirect reflection about the nature of infancy. Just as a newborn is attached to a mother whose functioning can seem emotionally indistinguishable from its own, so too is the ego function of consciousness similarly attached to a remnant of this primary relationship. While the union is too archaic to be remembered, it nevertheless becomes embedded in the developing personality.

The unperceived part of the ego to which consciousness is attached can be said to be derived, at least in part, from this primordial relationship with the mother. The infant experiences the ego support provided by its relationship with its mother as having its derivation within the realm of its narcissistic orbit. Because of this, the attachment to the mother becomes internalized as a part of the ego that is unperceived. The part of the ego that is not perceived is that part that existed before the achievement of the

---

[1]Cited in Kohut (1966, p. 251).

7

developmental capacity to objectify the mother *as an object* in a mentally experienced representational world. This is what could be called a pre-object relationship, a normal state of earliest development in which the baby concretely experiences its mother's functioning as part of itself. From the perspective of pre-object relatedness the mind–body problem in philosophy is an inevitable result of a developmental given, the outcome of the mother's mental mediation of the infant's physical distress, of the harmony or disharmony of her mind with the experiences of the baby's body.

The intrasystemic perspective of pre-object relatedness contributes to psychoanalytic conceptions of primary identification, introjection, affect regulation, psychic structure formation, and the reciprocal primal relatedness that forms the archaic substrate of the psychoanalytic situation. The infant's primitive internalizations of its experience of the infant–caregiver relationship pattern (Emde, 1988a) lays the groundwork for mental health or structural deficiency and developmental arrest (Osofsky and Eberhart-Wright, 1988). These relationship patterns are precocious; they are present at, or even before, birth (Piontelli, 1992); begin to be more fully internalized in infancy; exert a strong influence on all subsequent development, and are activated by similar contexts of relatedness throughout life (Emde, 1988a, b). Such a perspective enables the psychoanalytic clinician to bring his or her understanding of the very early development of object relationships to bear on the pathology of self-experience, and vice versa. Because pre-object states are by their nature preverbal, sensorimotor, affective, and concrete, this study addresses areas of experience that are to some extent elusive in a psychotherapeutic enterprise whose theory of technique idealizes the centrality of verbal association and symbolic communication. Yet the value of the attempt, despite its elusiveness, may be a better understanding of what Freud referred to as "the unperceived core of the ego" to which we are all ineluctably attached.

The attempt to better understand the link of this unperceived core of the ego to infancy is by no means new. As early as 1940, D. W. Winnicott insisted at a scientific meeting of the British Psycho-Analytical Society that "there is no such thing as an infant." He meant that an infant could not exist without maternal care, could not properly be thought of as a psychological unit when studying its emotional development, and could only be considered in the context of its caregiving surround. This disarmingly simple statement, first mentioned in his writings only in a footnote (Winnicott, 1960a), was a direct challenge to the defining emphasis on intrapsychic processes prevalent in both the Freudian and Kleinian ego psychologies of the time. Winnicott believed this distortion was inadvertently introduced because to that point most of the hypotheses concerning infants were reconstructions derived from adults in analysis. Unit status could be taken for granted in adults. The central theme in many of Winnicott's papers was a recurring one: the autonomous maturational potential of an individual could only be realized in the context of good-enough support from his or her environment. René Spitz's (1945) studies of the disastrous consequences of maternal deprivation to infants glaringly bore out the truth of Winnicott's observation.

Slowly, psychoanalysis—supported by many years of contributions from the fields of child analysis, object relations theory, self psychology, attachment theory, and infant developmental research—has begun to broaden its study of unconscious conflict from the exclusive perspective of a drive-oriented one-person psychology. Nowadays the intrapsychic sources of conflict and anxiety are more likely to be understood in the "new context" (Modell, 1984) of a two-person field. Stolorow (1991) exemplifies this change in psychoanalytic outlook when he writes that "intrapsychic phenomena must be understood in the context of the larger interactional systems in which they take form" (p. 176).

Such a shift in viewpoint necessitates a reexamination of the foundations of psychoanalytic thought, especially as it pertains to our conceptualizations about the sources of ego defense, articulated in Freud's theory of signal anxiety. Freud set forth this theory, still central to the psychoanalytic understanding of psychopathology, in 1926, radically altering his previous economic hypothesis of affects in the process. According to the newer theory, that part of the ego that constantly scans both the external and internal environment, sensing the imminence of danger, sends an affect-laden signal of anxiety. The part of the ego that receives and understands this signal as a sign of distress defensively alters its behavior in order to protect itself from the anticipated danger.

In ways that I will discuss more fully, the capacity of the ego to send as well as to receive its own behavior-modifying danger signals derives from residues of the infant–mother relationship.

The gradual internalization of these interactions from each individual's prehistory—which the infant is prestructured to forge—determines, to a large degree, the later capacity or incapacity to regulate his or her own affects. These earliest internalizations are at once archaic, psychosomatic, and presymbolic and predate the capacity to objectify the mother's presence in a mentally constituted representational world. Based as they are on need, such early experiences precede the instinctual relationship with the object (Gaddini, 1992). Such pre-object interactions are at first characterized by the intermodal transfer of emotional signals from infant to mother as well as the reciprocal transfer of adaptive emotional "shapes" and concrete regulatory functions from mother to infant. Pre-object relations are the self-structuring precursors for the development and maturation of self-identity, cognitive and emotional functioning, and differentiated object relationships. While pre-object relations likely begin even prior to birth, they persist into adulthood as the psychosomatic background of self-experience, as the "Erlebnis" or subjective sensation of one's own ego, mentioned in passing by Freud and first explored in detail by Paul Federn (1952). As Josephine Klein succinctly states in the title of her 1989 paper, "the vestiges of our early attachments become the rudiments of our later well-being."

A BRIEF DESCRIPTION
OF FREUD'S ANXIETY THEORIES

In his second theory Freud postulated that anxiety begins in utero. He did not, however, come to this understanding initially. His earlier theory of anxiety was linked to the psychic economics of pleasure. When he later retracted this theory, he wrote in retrospect: "I believed I had put my finger on a metapsychological process of direct transformation of libido into anxiety. I can now no longer maintain this view. And, indeed, I found it impossible at the time to explain how a transformation of that kind was carried out" (1926, p. 109).

In his struggle to work out a more accurate formulation, Freud gradually altered the foundations of his thinking about anxiety in particular and affects in general. He asserted that at its earliest and most primitive level of functioning the human organism endeavors to reduce unpleasurable stimulation from either external or internal sources to its lowest possible level and that with the aid of its mother's affect-buffering actions the infant creates a stimulus barrier (Freud, 1920) to external stimuli. In relation to inner stimuli, the infant's central motivating force was seen to be drive discharge, which would lead progressively to the buildup of unpleasurable tension if it could not be accomplished. Freud initially conceptualized the mother nonspecifically as the object through which drive reduction was achieved and the pleasure principle maintained.

In 1914, Freud linked his theory of anxiety and his emerging conception of a compulsion to repeat. In "Remembering, Repeating and Working Through," Freud made it clear that many individuals are able to give expression to their repressed memories only through external acts. For individuals who are unable to consciously remember, discharge is accomplished behaviorally, through repetition in motor activity, rather than psychologically, through trial action in memory or fantasy.

In "Inhibitions, Symptoms and Anxiety" (1926), one of his last major works, Freud moved the nature of primitive neonatal adaptive needs to a central role in his evolving theory of anxiety. This considerably more detailed and microscopic model asserted that not merely behavior but also affect states are repeated. Anxiety, in particular, was described as being the ego's repetition of a past affect associated with the memory of a danger situation: "Affective states have become incorporated in the mind as precipitates of primeval traumatic experiences, and when a similar situation occurs they are revived like mnemic symbols" (p. 93).

According to Freud, anxiety generated by any situation experienced as similar to that which was traumatic in the past signals the potential of danger to the ego, which then institutes defensive measures. Clarifying the relationship of symptom formation to anxiety, Freud made clear that symptoms are not created in order to avoid anxiety but in order to avoid the *danger situation* whose presence the anxiety signals.

Freud established a developmental line for prototypical danger situations. The developmental line begins with the danger for the fetus of birth. It progresses through the danger for the infant of psychical helplessness, the danger for the young and dependent child of loss of the object, the danger of castration for the child in the phallic phase; and the danger of punishment (i.e., fear of the superego) for the latency-age child. Freud's theory implies that, as one matures, one's perception of the nature of anticipated danger becomes increasingly associated with one's relations with loved and hated others and with the mental representations of those object relationships.

FOUR ASPECTS OF THE PRE-OBJECT DIMENSION OF SIGNAL ANXIETY

In an important passage in "Inhibitions, Symptoms and Anxiety" Freud (1926) wrote:

> Anxiety is seen to be a product of the infant's mental helplessness which is a natural counterpart of its biological helplessness. The striking coincidence by which the anxiety of the new-born baby and the anxiety of the infant in arms are both conditioned by separation from the mother does not need to be explained on psychological lines. It can be accounted for simply enough biologically; for, just as the mother originally satisfied all the needs of the foetus through the apparatus of her own body, so now, after its birth, she continues to do so, though partly by other means. There is much more continuity between intra-uterine life and earliest infancy than the impressive caesura of the act of birth would have us believe. What happens is that the child's biological situation as a foetus is replaced for it by a *psychical object-relation* to its mother. (p. 138; emphasis added)

Thus Freud replaced an exclusively economic theory of anxiety formation, in which anxiety is considered as being secondary to the impeding of drive discharge, with the beginnings of an object relations theory. In this new view, anxiety is a dynamic generated by the ego's conflictual relations with its objects, both before and after the infant's achievement of the ability to consciously discern the separate existence of its objects or of itself.

Implied in Freud's statement is a model of affect regulation based not only on a developmental theory of internalized object relations but also on a theory of pre-object relations. Freud (1926) asserts that archaic emotional experiences serve as the seeds for normal or pathological emotional development and asks us to imagine the possibility of fetal feeling-states. He places these prerepresentational experiences on a developmental line leading from an intrauterine state to birth, from birth through the psychology of the earliest infantile helplessness, and from these inchoate neonatal affects to the capacity to utilize emotions for their signal qualities. Anna Freud (A. Freud, with J. Sandler, 1981) amended the theory of signal anxiety to describe how ego defenses can be initiated by unpleasure as well as anxiety, and Krystal (1988), modernizing the theory even further, showed convincingly that all affects can act as a signal. As the infant develops a state of subjective awareness of relatedness to a perceived external object capable of ameliorating unbearable affects, it develops the ability to intentionally signal that person for help. This interaction is ultimately internalized and culminates in the child's ability to recognize and regulate its own affects. In other words, the child becomes able to signal impending distress to itself and to respond to those signals with a self-soothing reaction.

Bion (1977), taking up the above statement by Freud, admitted that while there may never be a chance to know what a fetus thinks, "there is no reason why it shouldn't feel" (p. 514). He wrote:

> It seems to me that from a very early stage the relation between the germ-plasm and its environment operates. I don't see why it shouldn't leave some kind of trace, even after the "impressive caesura of birth." After all, if anatomists can say that they detect tumors which really derive from the branchial cleft,[2] well then, why should there not be what we would call mental vestiges or archaic elements which are operative in a way that is alarming and disturbing because it breaks through the beautiful calm surface we ordinarily think of as rational, sane behavior? (1977, p. 514)

Freud's theory describes the prerepresentational precursors of what later develop into the differentiated structures of self-representations and object representations. To clarify my discussion, I will separate Freud's description of signal anxiety into four components. These four components, described in Table 1.1, are perception, communication, reception, and mediation.

The successful initiation of defense by the ego operates to tone down and moderate the intensity of the affect signal, achieving a homeostatic equilibrium in which affect is tolerable and activating to the ego rather than overwhelming and disorganizing. In signal affect the four aspects of the self, being felt in concrete somatic terms, very likely represent the experiential remnants of a pre-

---

[2] The embryological vestiges of gills.

TABLE 1.1. The Four Components of Signal Anxiety

Component	Function
1. Perception	The ego recognizes a potential danger situation.
2. Communication	The ego sends a signal of anxiety to itself.
3. Reception	The ego receives the signal of danger.
4. Mediation	The ego institutes defensive measures whose aim is to reduce the potential danger and to regulate the experience of anxiety.

object relationship that existed prior to the infant's capacity to form stable mental representations, to consciously differentiate itself from its caretakers, and to sort out its mental from its physical experiences.

Pre-object relations antedate the development of the infant's capacity to internally represent constant, differentiated object relationships. The term *pre-object* is perhaps awkward and easily misunderstood by anyone not familiar with the particular psychoanalytic meaning of the term *object relationship,* which refers not to the actual relationship with another person but with the quality of the mental representation of that relationship. Tyson and Tyson (1990) stated that the problem with most psychoanalytic terms for earliest developmental experiences is that they imply little interaction between mother and infant. They suggested the term *primary reciprocity* to describe these earliest developmental experiences. Their term well describes my meaning, although it is less amenable to my goal of integrating a theory of "prepsychology" with current psychoanalytic object relations theory. I emphasize, therefore, that I do *not* mean that the baby in the pre-object state is unrelated to others or is autistic. I mean only that the pre-object baby is not yet aware of itself in relation to others in a stable, ongoing, cohesive, and internalized manner. In fact, *the pre-object state is an archaic form of reciprocal relatedness for which the baby is preadapted from birth but about which the baby cannot yet "think"*; it is a prestage of what the growing infant will later mentally represent as an object relationship.

An analogy would be the nature of our relationship to gravity prior to Newton's discovery of it. The people of that time were affected no less by the effect of gravity despite their science not yet encompassing the concept of gravity. They did not fly off into space; they were not like the cartoon coyote who after racing off the face of a sheer cliff in hot pursuit of a speedy desert bird does not plummet to the canyon floor until he realizes that he can fall. Similarly, the infant is no less affected by its relationships with its caretakers just because it is not yet capable of apprehending them in the sophisticated way that it will later be able to, namely, by carrying around stable mental representations of them inside itself for internal navigation and refueling. In this sense, the pre-object infant is attached to its caretakers as closely as the pre-gravitation-concept individual of Newton's day was anchored to the surface of the earth. In both cases a force not yet fully discovered is nevertheless continually active.

In this sense we can paradoxically think of infants as being vitally enmeshed in relatedness with others prior to the time they are actually object related. In the psychoanalytic sense of the term the mother is only an object as the baby's mental representation of her. According to J. Sandler (1987b),

> When we speak of cathexis of the external world, or of objects in that world, we mean the cathexis of representations within the ego, representations that have been built up by successive experiences of the real world; experiences, however, that represent reality as distorted by the child's intellectual limitations, by his memories, wishes, and defense mechanisms. (p. 4)

However, at the beginning of life the mother has not yet been fully differentiated from the ego and is only experienced as an object in the psychoanalytic sense retrospectively (Chasseguet-Smirgel, 1985b). Stern (1985) stated that the neonate experiences global amodal representations, "not sights and sounds and touches and namable objects" (p. 51). Emde (1983) described the first weeks of life as essentially "prerepresentational," and Brazelton and Cramer (1990) claimed that object permanence does not occur until four to five months of age. E. Gaddini (1969) described the earliest psychic operations as based on imitation of physical perceptions rather than on higher-level mental operations such as introjection and identification, both of which require at least rudimentary mental representation.

Stern (1983) argued cogently that neonates have an innate prestructured capacity to discriminate between self and others but nevertheless distinguished between the infant's early *schema* of self and others and its later *representations* of self and object. It is only when the infant's sensorimotor schemata of others become stable mental representations capable of symbolic transformation that it is possible to conceive of them as objects in the psychoanalytic sense. Thus, while infants may possess the innate cognitive capacity to distinguish between sensorimotor experiences of self and other, this capacity may paradoxically be promoted and supported by the unperceived and largely undifferentiated holding environment that the good-enough mother naturally provides. It is this earliest relationship of an infant with its mother that supports the baby's capacity to express its prestructured developmental capacities. Describing this "primary relatedness," Kinston and Cohen (1986) stated that it is "an environmental complement to the individual and so cannot be internalized" (p. 343). Discussing what they call the "primary relationship," de Jonghe, Rijnierse, and Janssen (1991) stated the following:

> The primary relationship is an object relation with a narcissistic relatedness, i.e., with a narcissistic libidinal tie between a not-yet-subject and a pre-object, part-object, or self-object. We consider the term "object relation" unfortunate here for there is no object involved in it. "Pre-object relation" would be more accurate. (p. 700)

Psychoanalysts have developed the concept of *primary identification* to describe the nature of the infant's relatedness with its mother prior to the development of ego boundaries, which encompass the experience of subjective agency and an interior space with a personal internal representational world. The notion of primary identification is theoretically necessary in order to describe the nature of internalization prior to the infant's capacity to mentally represent the mother. Not everyone likes this way of conceptualizing the developmental prestages of identification, however. Arlow (1986), for example, argued that the phrase *primary identification* is inherently contradictory. He began by defining identification as a specific way "that an individual, consciously and/or unconsciously, thinks of himself as being, acting or playing the role of some other person" (p. 245) and on this basis drew the following conclusion:

It is misleading to speak of "primary identification," of identification before the individual has reached the stage of self–object differentiation. There are undoubtedly certain biologically determined, inborn, imitative responses that have had survival value from an evolutionary point of view. To the outside observer of behaviour, these actions may seem like identifications. They are imitative reflexes, responses to specific perceptual configurations. They correspond to neither the psychological function nor the meaning of identification that applies after the stage of object constancy and self–object differentiation has been achieved. There is no evidence that they have ideational content that leaves any persistent memory trace. (p. 245)

There is, however, a tautological aspect to Arlow's argument. Certainly, by defining identification as pertaining solely to a phenomenon of the representational world, it follows that identification *so defined* cannot exist prior to the development of that representational world. However, by thinking of identification so narrowly we run the risk of leaving no room to consider the compelling questions about the nature of the developmental precursors of identification. If Stern is correct in supposing that neonates are capable of primitive distinctions between schema of self and of others, then primary identification would indeed be possible. While not identification proper, these distinctions can be conceived of as suggesting identification-*like* responses, which, increasingly, infant observation research convincingly demonstrates *do* have a decisive effect on mental and emotional development despite their lack of symbolic ideational content. Stern (1985b) described the ability of infants to represent information preverbally as representations of interactions that have been generalized (RIGs). He suggested that the infant's ability to abstract and represent interactive experience as RIGs occurs "much earlier" than 10 months and claimed that "RIGs can thus constitute a basic unit for the representation of the core self. RIGs result from the direct impress of multiple realities as experienced, and they integrate into a whole the various actional, perceptual, and affective attributes of the core self" (p. 98).

As early as 1952, Greenacre described how primal emotional experiences patterned later biological development:

Variations in the birth process may . . . increase the (organic) anxiety response and heighten the anxiety potential, causing a more severe reaction to later (psychological) dangers in life. Painful or uncomfortable situations of the earliest postnatal weeks, before the psychological content or the means of defense have been greatly elaborated, would similarly tend to increase the organic components of the anxiety reaction. (p. 53)

Developmental research has described how the biological and psychosomatic functioning of the infant is partially determined by an internalization of experiential factors. Blank (1976) cited numerous studies documenting the slow rate of development in institutionalized children, the variability in developmental quotients within the infancy period, and changes in developmental progression when marked environmental restrictions exist. She claimed that these studies indicate that even "such basic development as sensorimotor functioning" is influenced by the environment and especially the infant's relationship with its mother or primary caregiver. Call and Marschak (1976) described the high degree to which the infant's reflex activities, including head movements, rooting behavior, and orienting behaviors such as flexion and extension, are influenced by the "style of care" offered by the parent. Wallerstein (1975), citing developmental studies that demonstrate that a mother's soothing efforts provide an infant with many more visual experiences than her neglect, claimed that "in the array of mothers . . . the outer reality (here, both the maternal reality and the outer visual perceptual reality) can be so crucially different for each child. . . . Small, and at times chance, variations in environment can thus have large developmental and behavioral consequences" (p. 432).

Bennett (1976) was unequivocal when he stated, "One source of confusion is to assume that early individual differences of 'temperament' are genetically based. . . . It is precisely some of these varieties of temperament that evolve out of the complex mother–child interchange during the first weeks" (p. 88). James (1972) insisted that "acquired constitution is not a foolish, paradoxical idea. Certain experiences in early life have the quality of ethological imprinting" (p. 439). These observations support the usefulness and validity of a psychoanalytic concept of primary identification as being a hallmark of the pre-object reciprocal relatedness of infant and parent.

CHAPTER TWO

Precursors
of Internalized
Object Relationships

THE PSYCHOANALYTIC CONCEPT of the object has acquired a contemporary meaning that is no longer grounded in the instinct theory from which it evolved. The object is no longer conceived of exclusively as the vehicle of instinctual gratification and discharge or as the energic investment of the mental images of other people. Object relations are now also thought of as crucial organizers of the emotional, cognitive, and psychosomatic needs of the infant, child, adolescent, and adult. While such needs may make themselves known in the form of wishes, these wishes need not be primarily instinctual in origin (Sandler and Sandler, 1978). This current understanding is a conceptual advance in one sense, but the psychoanalytic theory of object relationships still lacks cohesiveness about the developmental precursors of such integrated internal processes and the ways in which they develop. A plethora of competing developmental theories about the nature of the prestages of object relationships has emerged over the last 30 years. There is a recent trend, however, to forge a synthesis of what were thought of previously as discordant views, aided by the recent keen interest of psychoanalysis in infant observational studies. In this chapter I describe how the concept of pre-object relatedness lends itself to an effort to integrate a variety of views about how infants "internalize" the interactional successes and failures of the first weeks and months of their lives.

SPITZ'S CONCEPT
OF A "PREOBJECT" DEVELOPMENTAL PHASE

The term "preobject" was first advanced by René Spitz (1965) in his efforts to understand the smile response that develops at approximately two months of age. Spitz's observations indicate that the smile response emerges as an age-specific behavioral manifestation in 98 percent of infants between two and six months of age. Infants will smile at all human faces—friend or stranger, female or male, and regardless of race. After six months most infants reserve their smiles for those they are attached to; they no longer smile when a stimulus that previously elicited a smile is presented by a stranger. From his observations Spitz concluded that the smile response of the three-month-old infant is nonspecific and does not represent a true object relationship. An object relationship in the psychoanalytic sense is characterized by the experience of an ongoing relationship over time between the self and another person who is perceived as a separate individual. Spitz concluded that the smile of the three-month-old is elicited by a "sign Gestalt" of forehead, eyes, and nose, all in movement, and does not indicate recognition of a loved human partner.[1] This archaic form of relatedness does not, as such, constitute a whole object relationship but, rather, the precursor of an object relationship.

> If we related this finding to the system of psychoanalytic theory, it is obvious that the sign Gestalt is not a true object; I have therefore called it a *preobject*. What the infant recognizes in this sign Gestalt are not the essential qualities of the libidinal object; not the attributes that motivate the object to minister to the infant's needs, to protect and gratify him. What he recognizes during the preobjectal stage are secondary, external, unessential attributes. He recognizes a sign Gestalt, which is a configuration within the human face—not within a specific individual face, but within any face presented to him straight on and in motion. (Spitz, 1965, p. 91)

Spitz's use of the term "preobject" differs somewhat from the way I conceive of its usage here. Spitz used the term in a highly particular way, namely, to refer to a stage of development of circum-

---

[1] To support this conclusion Spitz demonstrated that a cardboard mask of a face is just as effective as a human face in eliciting a smile from a three-month-old.

scribed length between approximately two and six months. As I will elaborate further, I use the term in a far more encompassing sense to describe any of a variety of archaic forms of relatedness that are present at birth but persist throughout life. Pre-object relatedness, so conceived, persists in the background as the core of primary relatedness, the sense of "being there" and "being with" which accompanies all normative human experience.

Spitz thought of the preobject stage of development as the outgrowth of an earlier developmental phase he characterized as being "objectless." This notion appears to have been an effort by Spitz to make his observations consistent with Freud's theory of infantile development. However, the supposition of an objectless phase of development is misleading. First of all, more recent infant research demonstrates that neonates (and perhaps even fetuses) are highly aware of their surroundings, discriminating in their perceptions, and actively engaged with their caretakers and surroundings. Further, Spitz himself made clear that the neonate is intimately connected with its mother from birth on although it does not yet have the ability to endow stimuli with enduring meaning, that is, to know that its mother is its *mother*. This is not the same as autism or objectlessness. It is merely a primitive form of experience, which could not even continue to exist without enmeshment in the pre-object relatedness that is a prerequisite for life. While pre-object relatedness differs from more advanced "whole" or "true" object relationships and functions as a precursor to its development, it now appears that babies are never fully "objectless."

In addition, I postulate that pre-object relatedness is not vestigial, as Spitz thought, but is ongoing and continually structures all human relationships. Pre-object relatedness does not fade from existence with the advent of the capacity for differentiated object relationships but accompanies all object relationships as the affective, autonomic "core" that renders one's experience of self and others uniquely one's own. As Loewald noted, "Early levels of psychic development are not simply outgrown and left behind but continue to be active, at least intermittently, during later life including adulthood. They coexist, although overshadowed by later developmental stages, with later stages and continue to have their impact upon them" (1973, p. 81).

Because of these distinctions, as well as others that I describe throughout this book, I hyphenate pre-object to indicate my altered usage of the term. This hyphenation is consistent with Loewald's reintroduction of the concept, as when he asserted that "object-relations in the strict sense become constituted only on the level of the oedipal situation; prior to this stage in development, reality is *pre-objective*" (1973, p. 81; emphasis added).

REPRESENTATIONAL PRECURSORS

It is precisely because the infant's vital attachment to its mother predates the development of an internal representational world capable of consistently differentiating self and object, inside and outside, that psychoanalysts and developmental psychologists have asked themselves how the infant experiences this central relationship it cannot yet adequately represent mentally. In an attempt to address this question, a theory of mental operations that serve as precursors of representational thought has been evolving out of British object relations theory for over 30 years.

In one of Winnicott's (1963a) most far-reaching and yet most overlooked papers, "Communicating and Not Communicating Leading to a Study of Certain Opposites" there is an exploration of the change that comes about in the means of communication "*as the object changes over* from being subjective to being objectively perceived. . . . In so far as the object is subjective, *so far is it unnecessary for communication with it to be explicit*" (p. 182; emphasis in original). Winnicott asserts that the intercommunication between a neonate and mother is subtle and that a study of this communication would entail a study of the mother as much as the infant. However, once the infant becomes capable of perceiving the object objectively (e.g., is able to add object relating to pre-object relating), the infant becomes capable of both communicating and *not* communicating. Winnicott suggests that in health the core of the personality

> never communicates with the world of perceived objects, and that the individual person knows that it must never be communicated with or be influenced by external reality. . . . Although healthy persons communicate and enjoy communicating, the other fact is equally true, that *each individual is an isolate, permanently non-communicating, permanently unknown, in fact unfound.* (1963a, p. 187; emphasis in original)

Winnicott makes clear that it is the very centrality of this primitive but enduring "incommunicado element" that protects and makes possible the existence of a true self. He asserts that traumatic experiences that threaten the isolated core lead to the organization of primitive defenses that further hide the self's core from discovery and violation.

Bion (1962b), writing about the development of thought, postulated two prototypical elements of mental operations: alpha- and beta-elements. "Alpha-function," similar to what Piaget described as the semiotic function, operates on emotions and sensory experience to transform them into representation elements capable of being thought about, remembered, and dreamed. Beta-elements, in contrast, are more primitive mental operations that are not felt to be internal or mental but are experienced concretely. Beta-elements are not capable of representability and are thus unavailable for inclusion in thoughts, symbols, and dreams. Beta-elements, being "things-in-themselves," are not thought about as much as evacuated or manipulated; they are central in acting-out and in pathological projective identification.

> To learn from experience alpha-function must operate on the awareness of the emotional experience; alpha-elements are produced from the impressions of the experience; these are thus made storable and available for dream thoughts and for unconscious waking thinking. . . . Alpha-function is needed for conscious thinking and reasoning and for the relegation of thinking to the unconscious when it is necessary to disencumber consciousness of the burden of thought by learning a skill. (1962b, p. 8)

Bion contrasted alpha-function with beta-elements: "If there are only beta-elements, which cannot be made unconscious, there can be no repression, suppression, or learning. This creates the impression that the patient is incapable of discrimination. He cannot be unaware of any single sensory stimulus: yet such hypersensitivity is not contact with reality" (1962b, p. 8).

Ogden (1989a, b) wrote about "the most primitive state of being" as an "autistic–contiguous position," in which "raw sensory data are ordered by means of forming pre-symbolic connections between sensory impressions that come to constitute bounded surfaces. It is on these surfaces that the experience of self has its origins" (1989b, p. 49). Tustin (1990) described the normal earliest state of existence as an "auto-sensuous" state in which "all the senses are ready to be active; the responses are to alive and reciprocating objects that promote normal, on-going psychic development" (p. 218).

All these descriptions presume the very early capacity for at least rudimentary sensuous experiences of self and other prior to the development of a differentiated representational world. All of these authors are responding to the clear need for psychoanalytic theory to find better ways of conceptualizing the precursors of object relationships. I believe the concept of pre-object relatedness can be useful in the description and understanding of affect-regulating prerepresentational states in infancy and of similar experiences that characterize the primary relationship of patient and psychoanalytic therapist. In the following chapter I will describe how an understanding of the nature of pre-object relatedness helps to unify such disparate views of preautonomous affect regulation as Freud's theory of signal anxiety, Klein's theory of projective identification, and Kohut's theory of transmuting internalization.

INFANT–MOTHER INTERACTION

If, as Freud suggested, the affect development that begins as a fetus is supported after birth by the infant's interaction with its mother, then the gradual internalization of this relationship forms the core of what will later become the capacity to recognize and signal affects. The aspect of the ego that signals its distress corresponds to the infant who is experiencing some unpleasurable affect that threatens to "break through the beautiful, calm surface" (Bion, 1977) of its emotional tolerance. The aspect of the ego that receives the signal of distress derives from the mother who adaptively responded to her infant's suffering. It is controversial as to whether or not neonates are able to signal affects, and this is a question that further research will clarify (Emde and Buchsbaum, 1989). However, whether or not the neonate initially intends its affect to serve as a signal to the caretaker, it is likely that the caretaker *receives* the affect as a signal and responds accordingly. If all goes well, the physiological responses of the infant eventually become matched to the response patterns of the adult caretaker, for example, when the baby begins to sleep through the night. Sooner or later, affects become utilized by the infant for their signal functions and the mother's emotional response is echoed within the infant. How does this happen? Is the mother's response introjected, identified with, imitated, internalized, or matched to innate prestructured patterns?

Pre-Object Internalization

In the view of many, the neonate utilizes a prerepresentational form of thought. I use the term "representations" in the psychoanalytic sense, to convey enduring charged affective mental images of the self and significant others that are experienced as acting in a private internal space, or internal representational world. Prerepresentational experience would therefore be conceptualized as the necessary precursor to the later development of the capacity for representational thought. In this context *prerepresentational* does not mean "nonrepresentational"; indeed, significant infant research, which I will discuss in Chapter Four, suggests the possibility that certain amodal representational capabilities may be present at birth. Perhaps *proto-representational* would be a better word to use, since the prefix proto- means the "first" or the "earliest form of" something while the prefix *pre-* means "prior to" or "in advance of" something. In this sense *proto-object* might be a more accurate phrase than *pre-object*. The prerepresentational phase refers to an innate presentational capacity in human infants that precedes and makes possible the development of the semiotic and symbolic function necessary for *re*-presentation as conscious and unconscious thought. The prerepresentational state is characterized by sensorimotor processes, intermodal matching (Meltzoff, 1985; Meltzoff and Borton, 1979; Meltzoff and Moore, 1977, 1983a, b), and nonsymbolic, concrete, psychosomatic apprehension. The developmental line of pre-object relations progresses from prestructured sensorimotor schemata of self and other to the use of sensory shapes (Tustin, 1984), bounded surfaces (Anzieu, 1989; Bick, 1968; Ogden, 1989a, b), and hard objects (Kumin, 1978a; Tustin, 1980) for self-demarcation. Thereafter, the infant develops a beginning capacity to mentally represent objects in a partial way, although these part-objects are still fused with crude representations of the external object and/or one's own body. This is followed by the development of the capacity to create transitional objects and a transitional mental space as well as to utilize selfobjects in order to lend cohesion and positive affective coloring to one's own self-experience.

In contrast to the pre-object state of the infant, the personality attributes of the average mother include a structured representational world, an organized personality, a self-identity, empathic capacities, secondary process modes of thought, an adult ego capable of symbolic communication and synthetic thought, the capacity to recognize and regulate affects, the capacity to be preoccupied with the baby, and other primarily autonomous or secondarily neutralized ego functions. In other words, while the neonate's signal is originally prerepresentational, the mother is able to represent her infant's signal mentally and respond appropriately to it emotionally. At first the infant's signs of distress may have no intentionality, or specific cognitive meaning to the infant. Despite this, the infant's signs are given meaning by the parent. The infant's sign has symbolic significance as a signal of distress in the parent's emotional and representational world and enables the parent to adapt to the infant's needs. Because of this maturity gradient, any good-enough response from the adult caretaker to the distressed infant, whether behavioral, psychological, or affective, will tend to transmute (Kohut, 1971, 1977; Tolpin, 1971) the infant's sign into the precursors of a more neutralized, synthesized, symbolized, organized representational form that renders the infant better able to tolerate the now transformed affect. Just as primeval traumatic experiences serve as the substrate for later states of distress, primeval *adaptive* experiences during which the distressed infant is held and soothed by its caretaker serve as the neonatal substrate for the later development of a sense of well-being.

Loewald (1988), attempting to integrate a similar view with drive psychology, wrote:

> The first given to be assumed in psychoanalytic psychology is an interactional field, represented in its most primitive form by the infant–mother psychic matrix. What we call *instincts* in psychoanalysis . . . do not *ab initio* reside in an already separate psychic unit, the infant (or infant-self). In reference to the earliest stages of development, *instinct* (or *instinctual drive*) is a term for (interactional) psychic processes occurring in that matrix. Over the course of psychic differentiation—individuation—instincts become the motivational forces of an internal repertoire of the infant. The repertoire is by its origins

already marked by contributions from the motivational repertoire of the caretakers; it is not the manifestation of an innately autonomous infantile psyche. . . . *Primary narcissism* then is a title for the instinctual life of the mother–infant matrix. (pp. 32–33; emphasis added)

When the infant's caretakers act as an auxiliary ego to soothe and hold it, the infant internalizes the qualities and functioning of its caretaking environment. This will have an effect on how the infant perceives and experiences danger, tolerates affects, and develops a capacity to allay its own anxieties. The vicissitudes of such internalizations affect, for better or worse, the entire developmental line of ego formation, including such effects as the differentiation of mental ego from body ego and ego from id, the formation of an internal representational world; the generation of an ego boundary and the demarcation of self-representations from object representations; the establishment of secondary process thought and the reality principle; and the operation of the ego's adaptive and defensive activity, synthetic function, drive neutralization, sublimation, creativity, and secondary autonomy.

The outcome of pre-object internalization structures and conditions development after the achievement of "stable" self–object differentiation and in fact extends throughout one's lifetime. Tolpin (1971) pointed out the role of internalization of the mother's affect-regulating capacities in the development and outcome of stranger anxiety and the use of transitional objects. Another relatively early example of the developmental line of the affect-regulating pre-object activity of the infant–mother pair is the "appeal cycle," noted in an observational situation during the second year of life by Settlage and his coworkers (Settlage, Bemesderfer, Rosenthal, Afterman, and Spielman, 1988):

> The mother's diminished availability to her child . . . caused *every child* to evidence difficulty in maintaining independent functioning. Typically, the child at first appears to accept the diversion of the mother's attention and is able to function independently, engaging in self-initiated play and exploration. There then appear behavioral signs of mounting distress. This distress suggests the beginning failure of self-regulation and adaptation, and the need for assistance from the mother. For a time the child appears to struggle with this need. Eventually, the child makes a pointed appeal to the mother. The mother responds. The ensuing interaction relieves the child's distress

and, by inference, reestablishes self-regulation. The child returns to independent activity. After a time, distress is again evident and the cycle is repeated. (pp. 1–2; emphasis added)

Settlage et al., observing 12-to-24-month-olds in a clinical situation designed to test Mahler's concepts of separation–individuation, noted manifestations of the appeal cycle in all of the children in their study. Their observation that the appeal cycle is already in operation during the beginning of the second year of life suggests that the behaviors noted do not develop during the second year of life in response to phase-specific separation–individuation issues but, rather, evolve out of earlier pre-object developmental processes.

Pre-Object Affect Regulation

The affect-regulating functions provided to the pre-object infant by the mother eventually pattern the later development of affect-signaling and affect-regulating capacities of the mental apparatus in a number of other ways as well. Because signal affects develop prior to the time when an infant can reliably differentiate self from object images, all four aspects of the signal relationship are experienced as part of the self, a hallmark of pre-object functioning. This pre-representational internalization becomes part of the developing core of the infant's mental and body ego, affecting its psychosomatic functioning as well as its inborn capacity for affect generation and regulation (Taylor, 1987, 1992, 1993). In this way of thinking, one of the earliest functions of affect is as the infant's signal of distress *to* its mother and one of the earliest functions of the development of intrapsychic defense is to mimic within the self the affect mediation and affect tolerance that originally were provided *by* the mother. In particular, this means that *the self develops a pre-object relationship with those aspects of its own ego that have internalized the mediating functions of its original mothering objects.*

The ego function that receives and responds to the danger signal derives primarily from the internalization of the affect-regulating interaction of infant and mother that was experienced by the neonate as part of itself. One cannot soothe oneself in the absence of the stable internalization of that interaction. The baby's developing ability to integrate internal or external stimulation in a way that is not overwhelming or traumatic contributes to the development of a background feeling within the ego that Sandler (1960a) called "the background of safety." The development of this ability depends on a complex interaction of the genetic attributes of the infant and the quality of the support the infant receives from its mother. This observation has consequences for both normal development as well as for psychopathology. Settlage et al. (1988) described the changes in adaptive ego functioning and regulatory capacities of the rapprochement-subphase children once their mothers' attention was diverted for a while. The children showed mounting signs of distress, including making loud noises, exhibiting deterioration in motor control (manifested by uncharacteristic clumsiness), and thumb sucking. Kohut (1977), describing adult patients, described how the cohesive sense of self is undermined by the perceived loss of the narcissistic attachment to others who are felt to provide regulatory support.

Marian Tolpin's (1971) classic paper "On the Beginnings of a Cohesive Self" was one of the first to consistently describe the acquisition of self-soothing mental structures through the internalization of the mother's functions as a soother of the infant. Tolpin focused on the role of the transitional object as the concrete embodiment of a transitional selfobject representation of the mother's affect-buffering interactions with the infant and concluded that the vital self-soothing functions are internalized because of the "optimal frustration" of the separation–individuation phase, during which the infant replaces the lost symbiotic attachment to its mother's auxiliary ego support through "transmuting internalization." Tolpin predicated the crucial internalization on the exigencies of the separation–individuation phases:

> When the infant has learned that his mother's activities prevent the traumatic state, and that his distress signals directed to her have the same effect, the psyche has taken "a first great step forward" and is prepared for the beginning internalization of the mother's anxiety-reducing function. These internalizations provide the structural basis for the "transition" from automatic to signal anxiety. (1971, p. 33)

But how does the infant "learn" that the mother's activities prevent the traumatic state without having *already* begun to internalize her soothing functions? Accordingly, I suggest that the crucial internalizations occur significantly earlier than Tolpin postulated and that they emerge autonomously (e.g., not necessarily related to optimal frustration but to the innate nature of pre-object relatedness) and begin at or before birth. Such internalizations make the separation–individuation phase possible, not the other way around. The gradual accretion of autonomously occurring pre-object internalizations originating with earliest development renders the baby's relinquishing of the symbiotic attachment to its mother possible (that is to say, *tolerable*) to the infant's mind in the first place.[2]

Broucek (1979) set forward the notion that the development of a core sense of self is related to the infant's growing sense of agency and "efficacy." The infant experiences elation when it discovers that the behavior of exterior events is contingent upon its actions. Correspondingly, the infant feels crushed when it feels "unable to influence, predict or comprehend an event which [it] expected on the basis of previous experience to be able to control or understand" (p. 315). It follows that when the mother's response to the infant's sign of distress has been sufficient to provide adequate affect regulation and drive neutralization, the sign is extinguished and emotional equilibrium is created or restored. This occurs at least in part because of the reassurance that is created in the infant by its ability to control its own distress through the use of the mother and the omnipotent illusion she mediates as auxiliary ego. Winnicott (1971a) wrote cogently and eloquently about precisely this use of the object by the infant and the mother's role in the maintenance of this necessary, phase-appropriate illusion.

While psychoanalytic authors tend to describe infant–caretaker interaction producing affect regulation in terms of projective and introjective processes, these are by no means the only ways to describe these phenomena. For example, theorists from the ethological attachment model (Ainsworth, 1962, 1969, 1973, Ainsworth, Blehar, Waters, and Wall, 1978a, b; Bowlby, 1951, 1958, 1969, 1973, 1980, 1989; Lamb, 1978, 1981; Lamb and Easterbrooks, 1981) described similar processes in a more biobehavioral language. According to Lamb (1981):

---

[2]In Chapter Four I discuss the concepts of intermodal matching and intermodal exchange, which, when integrated with current psychoanalytic conceptions of symbiotic attachment, lead to a richer understanding of the earliest modes of infant–mother attachment.

Human infants are biologically predisposed to emit signals (e.g., cries, smiles) to which adults are biologically predisposed to respond. When adults consistently respond promptly and appropriately to infant signals, the infants come to perceive the adults concerned as predictable and reliable. This perception assures the formation of secure infant–parent attachments. . . . In contrast, when adults do not respond sensitively, insecure attachments result, and when they respond rarely, no attachments at all may develop. (p. 461)

Brothers (1989), citing evidence from comparative primatological studies that supports the idea that "sophisticated social communication is a hallmark of primate evolution" noted that "studies of human and nonhuman primate infants reveal the presence of innate and early responses to facial expression" and that "the phenomenon in man appears to be a product of *both species evolution and individual history*" (p. 17, emphasis added). While attachment theory has its own language and conceptual framework, its major emphasis on the signaling behavior of the infant and the optimal receptiveness of the adult who regulates infant affects and attachments appears to be congruent with the same emphasis found in psychoanalytic developmental psychology.

In fact, such congruence can be found among diverse psychoanalytic points of view as well, despite the tendency for the adherents of those views to emphasize their theoretical differences. In Chapter Three I discuss the centrality of the metaphor of the infant's signal of its distress to its mother and the mother's attuned responsiveness in classical, object relations, Kleinian, and self psychological theory.

Signal Anxiety and Environmental Mediation

A S THE INFANT'S EGO begins to develop signaling and receiving functions, these new capabilities assist in affect development. According to Krystal (1988, 1990), affect development includes the differentiation, tolerance, symbolization, and desomatization of affects. The infant becomes a more organized and communicative partner in the ongoing affective dialogue with its caregiving parent. Ideally, this increased emotional comprehensibility of the infant enables the parent to provide more specific adaptation to the infant's need and reduces the total amount of caregiving required. This is so in part because of the increasing achievement of functional independence of the now internalized affect-signaling and affect-regulating capacities of the infant.

But how does such signaling and subsequent internalization occur? This chapter and the next address this question. It is easy enough to understand how the caretaker's good-enough response to the signs that her infant is physically agonized or emotionally overwhelmed would lead to a reduction in the infant's distress, but it is more difficult to follow the steps by which the capacity for signal anxiety develops (or fails to develop) out of the successes and failures of the parent's earliest mediation[1] of affects. How does a self-caring response based on an internal replication of the model provided by the caretaker become part of the infant's mental and emotional repertoire for recognizing and responding to its own affects as signals?

In this chapter I discuss how an understanding of the concept of pre-object relatedness enables a synthesis and reinterpretation of seemingly disparate psychoanalytic theories. While the backgrounds of classical psychoanalysis, British object relations theory, and self psychology are often considered to be competing theoretical orientations, I hope to show that, at least in their consideration of the development of affect-regulating capacities in the infant, they share significant similarities that enable the formulation of bridging hypotheses. In the Chapters Four and Five I will describe the usefulness of infant research on intermodal matching in better understanding the nature of preverbal elements of the psychoanalytic situation.

FOUR STAGES OF SIGNAL ANXIETY

The preceding chapter discusses how the four stages of signal anxiety—perception, communication, reception, and mediation— also describe the normal affect-regulating interaction between the distressed infant and its soothing mother (Table 3.1). I concluded that this similarity was not a coincidence but a result of the pre-object, affect-regulating relationship of infant and mother that serves

---

[1]I borrow the word *mediation* in this book from Hans Loewald's (1960) paper "On the Therapeutic Action of Psychoanalysis," where he wrote the following:

> The parent ideally is in an empathic relationship of understanding the child's particular stage in development, yet ahead in his vision of the child's future and mediating this vision to the child in his dealing with him. This vision, informed by the parent's own experience and knowledge of growth and future, is, ideally, a more articulate and more integrated version of the core of being that the child presents to the parent. This "more" that the parent sees and knows, he mediates to the child so that the child in identification with it can grow. The child, by internalizing aspects of the parent, also internalizes the parent's image of the child—an image that is mediated to the child in the thousand different ways of being handled, bodily and emotionally. (cited in Loewald, 1980, p. 229)

More recently, Kinston and Cohen have also used the concept of emotional mediation in a central way in their theory of primal repression (Cohen and Kinston, 1983; Kinston and Cohen, 1986). I prefer *mediation* in some ways to similar terms, such as *holding* (Winnicott), *containing* (Bion), *metabolizing* (Langs), *role responsiveness* (Sandler), *selfobject* (Kohut), *anaclitic object* (Freud), *auxiliary ego* and *need-satisfying object* (A. Freud), because the term *mediation* is both descriptive and nonsectarian. However, I use all of these terms more or less interchangeably throughout this book.

as a pre-stage for the development of the ego's capacity for internalized affect regulation. The hallmark of this ability is the eventual development of the normal capability to signal affects. Once the interaction becomes internalized the baby becomes better able to intentionally communicate its needs to its caretakers. But more importantly, the baby becomes better able to respond adaptively to its own signs of distress. While signal anxiety takes places intrapsychically it derives from the pre-object interaction of the infant with its mother's emotional support and thus results in a similar intrasystemic interaction of one part of the ego with another. What was once the mother's ability to understand and mediate the nature of her baby's distress and to respond to it in a good-enough manner becomes transformed, as the baby matures, into what Freud called signal anxiety, the baby's increasing ability to recognize its own discomforts and to calm itself.

Recent psychoanalytic infant research, interpreting new data from a variety of research disciplines, has challenged the previously held notion that the neonate is not emotionally aware of or engaged with its caretakers. According to Emde and Buchsbaum (1989):

As knowledge accumulated concerning the young infant's complex organization, more research attention became devoted to effects of

TABLE 3.1. Four Stages of Affect Regulation

	Developmental model (infant–mother)	Freud's model (ego–ego)
1. Perception	Infant becomes emotionally distressed.	Ego perceives a potential for danger.
2. Communication	Infant displays unpleasurable affects and distressed motor behaviors.	Ego sends a signal of anxiety.
3. Reception	Mother receives infant's behaviors as a communicative signal.	Ego receives the affect signal.
4. Mediation	Mother adaptively attempts to soothe infant.	Ego institutes defensive operations aimed at reducing the experience of danger and the resulting anxiety.

social interaction originating within the newborn. It is not surprising that such effects are major, especially when one considers infant crying and its potential for initiating caretaking interaction. Today researchers are looking at both sides of a developing interactional system, with infant and caretaker being viewed simultaneously. Each partner is viewed as having separate competencies which affect the other's behavior and as initiating and reinforcing the behavior of the other. It is appreciated that the developmental process is *transactional*, with the behavior of each increasing in complexity over time. (p. 198; emphasis in original)

Shapiro and Stern (1989), addressing this same issue, asserted that the infant is fundamentally related to its objects from the beginning:

A first issue involves the growing evidence of developmental psychologists that the infant's perceptual apparatus is pre-wired or innately present from the moment of birth to form at least attentional ties with part-objects (the mother's face, voice, certain expressions).[2] These perceptual predilections toward the object, which foster object bonding, are present in the absence of any nurturing or drive-reducing experience with the object. They are constitutional. We view this evidence as in no basic way incompatible with psychoanalytic notions regarding the formation of object relations. If anything, it provides a firmer biological basis for the postulate of very early part-objects and in fact gives their early appearance a psychobiological "head start" toward becoming psychological entities rather than solely perceptual tendencies. (p. 288)

In arguing that the infant is fundamentally related to its mother in at least a rudimentary form from the very beginning, contemporary infant researchers support two of the once controversial ideas of the Scottish object relations theorist W. R. D. Fairbairn.

---

[2]It should be added that the infant also develops pre-object ties with parts of its own self; with its thumb, the interior of its mouth, its arms and legs, the pleased and pained sounds its voice makes, the tastes on its tongue, the smell of its excrement, its pleasure and unpleasure, its primary affects. The infant not only bonds to its mother, the infant bonds to its self. This relation of one's self to one's self as an object was first noted by Paul Federn (1952), who described the ego's simultaneous experience of itself as both subject and object as an irreducible paradox of existence. The relationship to the self as object develops into the foundation of the superego. Recently Bollas (1987), in particular, has studied this aspect of ego functioning.

Fairbairn (1952, 1954, 1958), challenging instinctual drive theory, argued that an ego is present from birth and that the infant's ego is fundamentally object seeking rather than pleasure seeking. Winnicott argued similarly when he contended that there is "no such thing as an infant," meaning that previous attempts to understand the infant as a unit without considering the contribution of the environmental provision by the infant's mother and other caretakers were fundamentally flawed. This orientation was further supported by many later studies confirming the catastrophic effects on babies of the loss of maternal caregiving.

John Bowlby (1951, 1958, 1969, 1973, 1980, 1989), a student of the British object relations theorists, later expanded this view when he formulated the beginnings of what later developed into attachment theory. Like Fairbairn, Bowlby challenged the notion, prevalent at the time, that object relations developed secondary to the gratification of instinctual drives. Bowlby considered attachment of infant and mother to be an innate, prepatterned behavior with adaptive and survival value for the human species. Other attachment theorists, observing human and animal infants, expanded our understanding of the crucial importance of the infantile tie to the mothering figure and the devastating effect that deprivation or disturbance of this attachment has (Ainsworth, 1962, 1967, 1969, 1982, 1985; Ainsworth et al., 1978a, b; Harlow and Zimmermann, 1959; Hinde and Spencer-Booth, 1971; Main and Stadtman, 1981; Main and Weston, 1982; Main, Kaplan, and Cassidy, 1985; Robertson, 1952).

Although studies of infant and primate attachment patterns have profound implications for psychoanalytic practice and psychoanalytic developmental theory, attachment theory is not in itself psychoanalytic (in the sense of being concerned with a depth understanding of the *subjective experience* of human attachments) in its outlook. Within psychoanalysis the two theoretical orientations that have been most singularly concerned with the development of human relatedness are object relations theory and self psychology. Familiarity with these perspectives leads to the discovery that each of their central paradigms of affect regulation parallels the four-stage process found in Freud's theory of signal anxiety. These organizing paradigms are the concept of projective identification in object relations theory and the concept of empathic attunement in self psychology. I now turn to a brief discussion of these concepts.

THE CONCEPTS OF PROJECTIVE
AND INTROJECTIVE IDENTIFICATION

Like most psychoanalytic ideas, the concepts of projective and introjective identification have gone through a complex development so that their current meaning differs considerably from the meaning originally assigned to them.

Melanie Klein

The related concepts of projective identification and introjective identification were originally described by Melanie Klein (1946). She considered projective identification to be a primitive intrapsychic fantasy employed during the first months of life in which "products of the body and parts of the self are felt to have been split off, projected into the mother, and to be continuing their existence within her" (1955, p. 310), with the fantasy that the object is identical to parts of the self modifying and controlling the experience of the object in the internal world. The modification and control of the object in fantasy helps the infant allay overwhelming early anxieties. While Klein believed that the actual behavior of the external object influences these fantasies (and vice versa), the primary emphasis in her work is on the economic relation of primitive mental processes with instinctual drives, particularly with the death instinct. Klein's theory, with its emphasis on the ongoing interaction of introjective and projective processes, provided the impetus for others to study the interaction of the infant's internal perceptual and fantasy world with the actuality of its external objects, but her own discussions of these issues are, for the most part, cursory.

D. W. Winnicott

D. W. Winnicott (1958a, 1965) alluded to the need to modify both Klein's and Freud's concepts of infant development, both of which he believed were overly focused on intrapsychic issues. He implicitly criticized both Klein's emphasis on the primacy of the infant's intrapsychic fantasies and Freud's emphasis on the primacy of the infant's instinctual drives. Winnicott argued that concepts relating to the infant's intrapsychic world were meaningless unless considered in relation to the actual quality of the environmental provision by the infant's mother. Asking himself whether the infant's ego should be thought of as strong or weak, he contrasted the relative ego strength of the baby who "gets support from the mother's actual adaptive behavior, or love, with the ego-weakness of the baby for whom environmental provision is defective" (1962, p. 63):

> In my terminology the good-enough mother is able to meet the needs of her infant at the beginning, and to meet these needs so well that the infant, as emergence from the matrix of the infant–mother relationship takes place, is able to have a brief *experience of omnipotence.* . . .
>
> So much difference exists between the beginning of a baby whose mother can perform this function well enough and that of a baby whose mother cannot do this well enough that there is no value whatever in describing babies in the earliest stages except in relation to the mother's functioning. When there is not-good-enough mothering the infant is not able to get started with ego-maturation, or else ego-development is necessarily distorted in certain vitally important respects. . . .
>
> At the stage which is being discussed it is necessary not to think of the baby as a person who gets hungry, and whose instinctual drives may be met or frustrated, but to think of the baby as an immature being who is all the time *on the brink of unthinkable anxiety.* Unthinkable anxiety is kept away by this vitally important function of the mother at this stage, her capacity to put herself in the baby's place and to know what the baby needs in the general management of the body, and therefore of the person. (1962, pp. 57–58; emphasis in original)

Implicit in Winnicott's theory is a conceptualization of early affect regulation along the lines of the four aspects of Freud's theory of signal anxiety, transposed to the infant–mother dyad. The infant

1. *Perceives* the unthinkable danger of annihilation and
2. *Communicates* this nameless dread to its good-enough mother, who
3. *Receives* the infant's distress because of her primary maternal preoccupation and
4. *Mediates* the baby's needs so that the unbearable can be borne and ultimately regulated internally by the infant.

Wilfred Bion

Wilfred Bion (1955, 1959) recognized the validity of the view that the infant and mother function as a system and significantly modified Klein's concept of projective identification in order to better take into account the interaction of the individual with the environment. He demonstrated that projective identification, far from being an exclusively intrapsychic fantasy, is an interactional process by which one individual is enlisted, and even unconsciously coerced, into playing a role in another person's fantasy. Bion traced this interaction to the earliest relationship of infant to mother and described projective identification as an early form of communication through which the infant is able to convey the nature of its overwhelming affects to its mother.

In Bion's description of projective identification the infant who is suffering from an unbearable emotion displays its distress to its mother in such a way that she can understand its communicated feelings. If she responds in the way that any "ordinary good-enough mother" (Winnicott, 1965) would, she does something to soothe the infant. The infant then feels better. According to Bion (1962b):

> Ordinarily the personality of the infant, like other elements in the environment, is managed by the mother. If mother and child are adjusted to each other, projective identification plays a role in the management through the operation of a rudimentary and fragile reality sense. . . . As a realistic activity it shows itself as behavior reasonably calculated to arouse in the mother feelings of which the infant wishes to be rid. . . . A well-balanced mother can accept these and respond therapeutically: that is to say, in a manner that makes the infant feel it is receiving its frightened personality back again but in a form that it can tolerate—the fears are manageable by the infant personality. If the mother cannot tolerate these projections, the infant is reduced to continued projective identification carried out with increasing force and frequency. (pp. 114–115)

Bion described projective identification in terms of the interplay between projective and introjective processes in the formation and maintenance of object relations. Bion's descriptions follow the pattern of the four aspects of Freud's theory of signal anxiety closely.

1. *Perception*: A part of the infant's budding self-repre-sentation that the infant senses is subject to an internal danger is externalized projectively.
2. *Communication*: The externalization subjectively rids the infant of the dangers associated with it and communicates this danger to the mother.
3. *Reception:* The infant's mother, who is attuned to her infant through what Bion calls a state of "reverie," senses the nature of her infant's discomfort and responds empathically with her vastly more integrated mental and emotional functioning. She acts like an "auxiliary ego" to help bolster her baby's efforts at damping down its overwhelming feel-ings.
4. *Mediation*: The infant then reinternalizes the formerly over-whelming feeling as something that can now be tolerated, as well as reinternalizing the previously projected aspect of its self-representation. The infant identifies with this aspect of itself as experienced by its mother. The baby "sees itself through its mother's eyes." As a result, the infant's self-rep-resentation now becomes more complete, splitting is re-duced, reality testing improves, drives are neutralized, and the synthetic function of the ego is supported. The infant's experience of the previously projected part of the self has become transformed by the effect of the mother's concern upon it.

Arthur Malin and James Grotstein

Malin and Grotstein (1966) clarified the particular interplay of projective and introjective mechanisms in projective identification, especially the role of what Melanie Klein first described as introjec-tive identification. In their view, projective identification is a normal process, existing from birth. They also described projective identifi-cation as a four-step process involving

1. The ego's *perception* of a danger requiring it to
2. Discharge "unwanted or disclaimed parts of the self" (p. 47), and *communicate* its distress by projecting aspects of the self-representation into the external object,

3. Enabling the *receiving* of the projected parts by the external object and
4. The reintrojection of the perceptual "alloy" of external-object-plus-projected-aspect-of-the-self that has resulted through the *mediation* of the external object.

Malin and Grotstein cited Loewald's (1960) paper on the therapeutic action of psychoanalysis, in particular Loewald's view that the patient in analysis achieves a "higher stage of organization" by way of his or her identification with the "organizing understanding" provided by the analyst. In their view, it is particularly the processes of projective and introjective identification that help explain how these higher levels of ego integration are achieved: "*It seems to us that it is only upon perceiving how the external object receives our projection and deals with our projection that we now introject back into the psychic apparatus the original projection, but now modified and on a newer level*" (p. 28; emphasis in original). Malin and Grotstein suggested that projective identification, thus conceived, "is one of the most important mechanisms by which growth and development take place through object relations. This mechanism can be described as one in which objects and associated affects are re-experienced on a new integrative level so that further synthesis and development will take place within the ego" (p. 31).

Thomas Ogden

Ogden (1979, 1982), expanding on the contribution of Malin and Grotstein, also conceived of projective identification as a four-step process involving a combination of projective and introjective mechanisms. He especially synthesized Malin and Grotstein's work with the earlier contributions of Klein, Bion, and Winnicott when he specified that projective identification is "a psychological process that is simultaneously a type of defense, a mode of communication, a primitive form of object relationship, and pathway for psychological change" (1979, p. 362). Ogden made the important point that the concept of projective identification can be considered entirely on its own merits and bears no essential relationship with Melanie Klein's theory or, for that matter, [with] that of any other school of psychoanalytic thought. In particular, there is no necessary tie between projective identification and the death instinct, the concept of envy, the concept of constitutional aggression, or any other facet of specifically Kleinian clinical theory or metapsychology. Moreover, there is nothing to tie the concept of projective identification to any given developmental timetable. (1979, p. 364)

Ogden demonstrated convincingly that all the concept of projective identification actually requires is that the individual (whether infant, child, or adult) be capable of a projective fantasy and of the specific types of object relationship involved in the reception and mediation of his or her distress.

Ogden's ideas epitomize the prevalent contemporary usage of the concept of projective identification (and the way in which I use the concept). In my view, *projective identification is a central developmental process by which adaptive responses may be elicited from others.* However, like any normal developmental process, projective identification may be pathologically distorted by a variety of factors, including innate biogenetic disturbance, internal conflict, trauma, or environmental deficit. It was perhaps because the first studies of projective identification focused on what would now be considered pathological projective identification that it was at first described as a vicissitude of the death instinct and thought to rely exclusively on splitting defenses. Clinically, projective identification as a defense was at first described with pejorative adjectives, such as "primitive," and its existence was attributed almost exclusively to patients exhibiting the most severe psychopathology. The adaptive use of projective identification in a variety of ordinary situations by well-functioning individuals was overlooked until relatively recently. Many psychoanalytic researchers now consider the developmental line of projective identification to be lifelong, normal, and adaptive, unless pathologically disturbed. Different aspects of this developmental view can be found in the works of such disparate writers as Wangh (1962), Langs (1977), Sandler (1987), Joseph (1987), and Kernberg (1987), among others. Rosenfeld (1987), to cite just one example, called projective identification a "benign and essential part of normal object-relating" (p. 161) and considered it to be the basis on which empathy develops.

THE CONCEPTS OF EMPATHIC ATTUNEMENT
AND TRANSMUTING INTERNALIZATION

Kohut's Contribution

Kohut highlighted a fundamental paradox that was implicit in the research of the ego psychologists, the British object relations school, the attachment theorists, and other infant researchers. He theorized that the seemingly autonomous functioning of one's self depended on an internalization of functions provided by others. These narcissistic functions provided by others were experienced as parts of the self. Such "selfobject" functions were conceived of as precursors of not yet existing psychological structures. According to Kohut (1971), narcissistic homeostasis ultimately depends on the gradual "transmuting internalization" of those ego functions originating from the object that supported the autonomous functioning of the self: "Just as the superego . . . is the massively introjected internal replica of the oedipal object, so is the basic fabric of the ego composed of innumerable (by comparison with the superego: minute) internal replicas of aspects of the *pre*oedipal object" (p. 47; emphasis in original).

In addressing Freud's question about how the drives are tamed, Kohut, like the object relations and attachment theorists before him, emphasized the vicissitudes of pre-object relations: "From the beginning, the drive experience is subordinated to the child's experience of the relation between the self and the self-objects" (1977, p. 80). The child's experience of this pre-object relationship depends inevitably upon the caretaker's ability to provide an environment capable of being attuned empathically to the child's needs. In a formulation owing much to the 1960 paper by Loewald cited earlier, Kohut (1977) asserted that the infant becomes able to regulate its own affects through a developmental process involving the internalization of qualities of its caretaker's more advanced mental functioning:

> The self-object, equipped with a mature psychological organization that can realistically assess the child's need and what is to be done about it, will include the child into its own psychological organization and will remedy the child's homeostatic imbalance through actions. . . . The child's anxiety, his drive needs, and his rage . . . have brought about empathic resonances within the maternal self-object. The self-

object then establishes tactile and/or vocal contact with the child (the mother picks up the child, talks to it while holding and carrying it) and thus creates conditions that the child phase-appropriately experiences as a merger with the omnipotent self-object. The child's rudimentary psyche participates in the self-object's highly developed psychic organization; the child experiences the feeling states of the self-object—they are transmitted to the child via touch and tone of voice and perhaps by still other means—as if they were his own. (pp. 85–86)

Kohut's thesis is also a view remarkably similar to that first set forward in the 1950s by Winnicott, with his emphasis on the good-enough mother's provision of a holding environment that is adapted to the infant's ego needs, and by Bion, with his descriptions of the role of projective identification in the infant's success in making its own affect states known to the mother and in its subsequent reinternalization of the mother's successes or failures in containing the affect within her reverie. In a passage that is similar to Malin and Grotstein's earlier formulation, Kohut (1977) wrote:

The relevant feeling states—either the child's own or those of the self-object in which he participates—in the order in which they are experienced by the self/self-object unit, are: mounting anxiety (self); followed by stabilized mild anxiety—a *"signal" not panic*—(self-object); followed by calmness, absence of anxiety (self-object). . . . It is the experience of this sequence of psychological events via the merger with the empathic omnipotent self-object that sets up the base line from which optimum (non-traumatic, phase-appropriate) failures of the self-object lead, under normal circumstances, to structure building via transmuting internalization. (pp. 85–87; emphasis added)

Kohut, too, like the object-relations theorists, asserts that affect regulation proceeds via the four-step process first described by Freud:

1. *Perception*: The baby experiences mounting distress because of archaic perception of its unmet needs.
2. *Communication*: The baby communicates its distress to its parent (who is experienced at meeting its selfobject needs).
3. *Reception*: The parent's soothing empathic response bolsters the child's ego functioning and affirms the child's sense of self.

4. *Mediation:* The parent's optimal responsiveness leads to increased calmness resulting from the child's internalization of the parent's soothing function. The child, through transmuting internalization, eventually internalizes the selfobject functions originally provided by the parents, although the need for selfobject support is never entirely relinquished. The nature of the internalization serves as a nidus for structuralization of subsequent autonomous strengths or weaknesses in the infant's developing capacity to regulate its own affects.

The similarities found in the conceptions of affect regulation between Freud's ego psychology, object relations theory, self psychology, and infant developmental research are striking. To be sure, the theories are not equivalent and contain important differences in emphasis, differences that receive far more attention in the psychoanalytic literature than do the similarities. For example, object relations theory emphasizes the role of externalization in affect regulation (and the Kleinians further highlight the function of inchoate aggression in such externalizations) while self psychology emphasizes the role of internalization (and tends to view aggression as being a secondary, adaptive reaction to faulty environmental attunement to developmental needs). Freud's theory emphasizes the intrapsychic aspects of affect regulation while the other theories are interactional in their emphasis. Yet, despite such differences, each conceives of affect regulation as a four-step process in which

1. Danger is *perceived,* anticipated or experienced.
2. A *communicative* signaling process is initiated.
3. The danger signal is *received.*
4. The danger is *mediated* by way of defensive operations whose aim is to reduce the level of experienced danger.

Taken together, psychoanalytic theories of anxiety present a developmental line of affect regulation progressing from early infantile affect mediation by the mother (Winnicott and Bion) to "transitional" and/or "selfobject" affect mediation during the latter part of the first and during the second year of life (Winnicott and Kohut), to progressively more internalized affect mediation by the ego during the rapprochement subphase of separation–individu-

TABLE 3.2. Psychoanalytic Schools as a Developmental Line of Affect Regulation

	Developmental Four stages of affect regulation (infant and mother)	Object relations Four stages of projective identification (external)	Self psychology Four stages of transmuting internalization (transitional)	Ego psychology Four stages of signal anxiety (internal)
1. Perception	Infant becomes emotionally distressed.	Individual experiences unthinkable anxiety, the experience of annihilation.	The self experiences mounting anxiety.	Ego perceives a potential for danger.
2. Communication	Infant displays unpleasurable affects and distressed motor behaviors.	The individual projects this overwhelming affect into the object and attempts to actualize the projection behaviorally.	It signals its distress to its selfobject	Ego sends a signal of anxiety
3. Reception	Mother receives infant's behaviors as a communicative signal.	The external object receives the projected parts.	The selfobject receives the signal of distress.	Ego receives the affect signal.
4. Mediation	Mother adaptively attempts to soothe infant.	On the basis of the external object's response, the individual reintrojects the object's adaptive response plus the projected aspect of his or her own self.	The empathic attunement of the selfobject leads to calmness and is eventually internalized via transmuting internalization.	Ego institutes defensive operations aimed at reducing the experience of danger and the resulting anxiety.

ation (Mahler) and during the oedipal phase and latency years (Freud's second theory of anxiety), and finally, to the "object removal" of adolescence (Katan). This progression is illustrated in Table 3.2.

While signal anxiety is thought of as an intrapsychic process and projective identification and transmuting internalization are thought of as interactional processes, the understanding that pre-object aspects of the infant–mother interaction are experienced as indistinguishable from one's self removes this artificial distinction between these concepts. Hartmann (1950b) made clear that certain ego functions not belonging to the constitutional inheritance of the individual can nevertheless develop functional independence of the interaction of the ego with the drives and external reality. Put another way, individual psychology develops in part from an internalization of the pre-object experience of a two-person matrix.

Chapter Four describes recent infant research that improves our capacity to conceptualize the means by which the preverbal infant and the mother exchange signals and affects in this two-person matrix. Chapter Five discusses the similar wordless means by which patient and analyst transmit their emotions to each other.

PART TWO

Intermodal Exchange

Intermodal Matching and Affect Transmission

PSYCHOANALYSTS were interested in whether and how emotions were transmitted from one person to another even before Freud wrote his 1925 addendum to "The Interpretation of Dreams." In that paper Freud made clear his conviction that one aspect of the dream work was the modification and transformation of affectively charged thoughts that had been "telepathically communicated" during the preceding day. Freud linked this activity to archaic mental activity, which he called our "basic language."[1] Since a developmental approach to the understanding of human motivation centrally organizes all psychoanalytic theories, an interest in the earliest forms of experience characterizes one of the leading edges of psychoanalytic research. Additionally, psychoanalytic practitioners are increasingly making use of a better understanding of the earliest developmental phases in order to adapt psychoanalytic treatment approaches to the needs of individuals who are regressed in the transference or are suffering from arrested early development. In this chapter I discuss infant research that I believe provides a new way of understanding the "basic language" of preverbal communication and apply the findings of this research to our comprehension of the way humans transmit and receive emotions without speech.

---

[1] A phrase Freud first noticed in Schreber's memoirs of his paranoid illness.

51

INTERMODAL MATCHING AND NEONATAL
REPRESENTATIONAL CAPACITIES

In a series of original and far-reaching papers Meltzoff and his coworkers challenged current conceptions of prelinguistic representational capacities and present compelling evidence that neonates have significantly more sophisticated representational competence than was previously thought (Kuhl and Meltzoff, 1982, 1984; Meltzoff, 1985, 1990; Meltzoff and Boran, 1979; Meltzoff and Moore, 1977, 1983a, b). Writing about early coordination of perceptual abilities across sensory modalities, Meltzoff (1985) stated that neonates "can represent adult behavior in non-modality specific terms that not only encode the event but also serve as the basis of self-action. On this view, visual perception and motor production are closely linked and mediated by a common representational system *right from birth*" (pp. 75–76; emphasis added).

The researchers reached this conclusion in a series of cleverly designed experiments. Meltzoff and Moore (1983a), studying imitation in infancy, discussed theorists who view the capacity for imitation to be the result of early learning and those, like Piaget, who assert that not all infant imitative behavior is the result of adult training. They noted that Piaget (1950, 1962) considered facial imitation to be a particularly important developmental milestone because, unlike manual and vocal imitation, the infant's response cannot be perceived with the same sensory modality as the model's. In other words, in facial imitation the infant must match an adult's facial gesture, which they can see, with their own facial imitation, which they cannot see.

Describing his experimental design intentions, Meltzoff (1985) wrote:

> In order to demonstrate imitation one must utilize what we have called a "cross-modal comparison." In this technique the infant is shown not only tongue protrusion but also another gesture that is produced (a) by the same experimenter, (b) at the same distance from the infant, and (c) at the same rate of movement. For example, one measures the infant's reactions to two facial gestures, such as tongue protrusion and mouth opening. If infants respond with more tongue protrusion to the tongue-protrusion display than to the mouth-opening display and,

conversely, respond with more mouth opening to the mouth display than to the tongue display, this would demonstrate imitation. This differential response could not be accounted for by a general arousal of infant motor activity by an adult face, nor even by some sort of specific arousal of feeding responses, because the same adult face is making similar oral movements in both conditions. If the infants respond differentially and in a way that is isomorphic with the adult's display, this is evidence for imitation. (pp. 65–66)

Safeguards were observed to maintain objectivity. Parents were not informed until after the experiment concluded that imitation was being studied. The experiments were designed in such a way that the experimenter could not alter the rhythm of his or her facial demonstration in response to the infant. After a 90-second period in which the adult maintained an emotionally neutral face, he or she then demonstrated one of four facial gestures four times in a 15-second period: lip protrusion, mouth opening, tongue protrusion, and sequential finger movement. The infant's reactions were videotaped and then scored by observers who did not know which facial gesture the infants had witnessed. In these laboratory studies of infant imitation Meltzoff and Moore (1977, 1983a, b) demonstrated that alert normal neonates under one month old (one only an hour old) can reliably imitate the facial gestures of adult testers (Figure 4.1). These findings have since been replicated by independent researchers utilizing similar research methodology.

This is a conclusion that calls into question many of the fundamental assumptions of learning theory, mainstream psychoanalytic theory, and Genevan (e.g., Piagetian) developmental psychology, all of which assert that such representational capacities cannot be achieved until many months later. For example, Piaget believed that only between 18 and 24 months could the baby begin deferred imitation. For Piaget (1962; Piaget and Inhelder, 1971, 1973), deferred imitation marked the beginning of the "semiotic function," the capacity to "internalize" one's imitative sensorimotor actions and to form "mental images of absent realities" (Meltzoff, 1985, p. 65). In contrast, Meltzoff and Moore (1977) suggest that "we must revise our current conceptions of infancy, which hold that such a capacity is the product of many months of postnatal development.

The ability [at birth] to act on the basis of *an abstract representation* of a perceptually absent stimulus becomes the starting point for psychological development in infancy and not its culmination" (p. 78; emphasis added).

Further, Meltzoff and Moore (1983a) argued that such early imitative capacity cannot be the result of an innate releasing mechanism, either, as described by the research of Lorenz and Tinbergen (Lorenz and Tinbergen, 1938; Tinbergen, 1951). The infants were able to imitate a whole range of motor actions, not

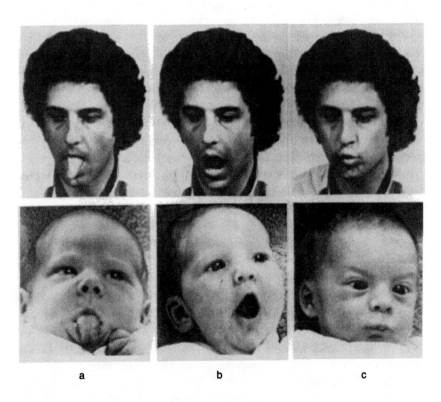

a   b   c

FIGURE 4.1.

Sample photographs from videotape recordings of two- to three-week-old infants imitating (a) tongue protrusion, (b) mouth opening, and (c) lip protrusion demonstrated by an adult experimenter. Reprinted with permission from Meltzoff and Moore (1977). Copyright 1977 by Andrew N. Meltzoff.

merely the single stereotypic fixed action patterns that classically characterize behaviors that are innately released. The infants did not produce perfect matching behaviors but instead were able to improve their responses over successive tries. Meltzoff and Moore (1983a) concluded that neither learning theory nor innate releasing mechanisms can account for this finding and suggested that neonates are able to generate equivalences between actions seen and actions done via the mediation of an innate representational system that allows them to "unite within one common framework their own body transformations and those of others" (p. 708). They supported this assertion in other, more complex, experiments that demonstrate the presence of what they called "intermodal matching."

One experiment (Meltzoff and Borton, 1979) demonstrated that month-old infants can visually identify complexly shaped objects they had actively explored with their mouths but had never before seen. Three experimenters were used to maintain objectivity. The first experimenter selected one of two pacifiers, one smooth and the other nubby, to give to the baby. A second experimenter placed the pacifier in the infant's mouth while hiding it from the baby's view. The baby was then turned to view replicas of the two pacifiers, which the first experimenter had positioned, while the second experimenter removed the pacifier from the infant's mouth. A third experimenter who was unfamiliar with both the shape of the pacifiers and with their left–right positioning monitored the pupils of the babies' eyes and recorded whether they visually fixated on one or the other pacifier. Half of the babies received the smooth pacifier and half the nubby one, half of the pacifiers were placed on the left and half on the right, and boys and girls were evenly distributed in each subgroup. Three-quarters of the babies tested fixated longer on the shape of the pacifier they were given than on the nonmatching shape. This clearly demonstrates the neonatal presence of intermodal coordination between the tactual and visual realms, the sophistication of which was previously thought possible only after considerable learning had taken place.

In another experiment a vowel sound (either "ah" or "ee") was played to an infant from a loudspeaker positioned midway between two television screens. On the screens were two filmed faces. One face made silent lip movements corresponding to the "ah" sound and the other face made silent lip movements corresponding to the "ee" sound. The oral movements on the screens were coordinated with each other. As in the previous experiment, the infants were videotaped and then scored as to which face they looked at longer. "Because the two faces were moving in perfect synchrony, there were no temporal cues. Because the sound emanated from a source equidistant from the two faces, there were no spatial cues. The only way the infants could solve the intermodal task was if they could recognize the correspondence [between the auditory and visual] speech information" (Meltzoff, 1985, p. 73). Seventy-five percent of the babies tested looked longer at the face matching the sound they heard, clearly demonstrating that they could match the information picked up by the eye and the ear. While the test was conducted with four-month-olds and so cannot exclude the effects of previous learned experiences, the tests do demonstrate that the capacity for intermodal matching occurs at a very young age and supports the findings of earlier studies by the same researchers.

On the basis of these experiments Meltzoff (1985) concluded as follows:

> First, this research suggests that newborns are not born with five separate and independent sensory channels. Rather, newborns initially bring to their interactions with people and things some basic ability to detect and utilize equivalence in information picked up by different sensory modalities. It is as if the perceptual modalities already "speak the same language" at birth. . . .
>
> Second, . . . it can be hypothesized that sensory-motor imitation may not be internalized to become mental imagery, as described by Piaget. On the contrary, there appear to be interesting representational capacities present at birth (which is not to deny significant development in them afterwards), and *it may be these very representational capacities that allow for imitation in the first place.* (p. 75; emphasis added)

Psychotherapists have long noted similar findings in adults and children. A patient of mine experienced hearing an accurate interpretation as a concrete physical sensation in her mouth. Furman and Furman (1984) described a latency age boy with deviant ego development who received from his teachers on his sixth birthday a gift of a set of rubber stamps for making a variety of images. The boy "opened the package and put the stamps in his mouth one by one. When asked what he was doing, he replied, 'I am looking at them' " (p. 423).

As early as 1937, Ella Freeman Sharpe offered the following account of intermodal matching in a patient:

> Colours in dreams are very important for one of my patients. I always ask for more details concerning any colour, and, in addition, if the colour is pertaining to material, I ask for details concerning the type of material. I have proved conclusively through this patient my surmise that both creative imagination and artistic appreciation are firmly rooted in the earliest reality experiences of taste, touch and sound. For this patient an oatmeal-colored material had a "crunchy" feeling and the "crunchy" feeling in her fingers always brought sensation in her teeth.
>
> A cherry-coloured silk will make her mouth water and she longs to put her cheeks gently on its surface. The range of colours for this patient are in terms of cream, butter, lemon, orange, cherry, peach, damson, wine, plum, nut brown, chestnut brown. Materials can be crunchy like biscuits, soft like beaten white of eggs, thick like cake. Threads can be coarse like the grain of wholemeal bread, shine like the skin of satin. I do not let any reference to colour or material or to dress escape me in the dreams this patient brings. (Sharpe, 1978, pp. 92–93)

AFFECT MATCHING

Meltzoff's research illustrates the infant's primary identity with its caregivers, an identity rooted in reality experiences. Infants are innately able to match themselves to their mothers across sensory modalities. Meltzoff and Moore (1992) concluded that the early imitation and sharing of behavioral states serves an identity function that enables young infants to differentiate and communicate with persons as opposed to things. Such abilities would also enable the infant to "mold" to the qualities of the holding environment in ways far deeper and more fundamental than mere postural molding. The normal infant develops an ability to mold itself not only to the shape of its mother's arms but also to her voice, her facial expression and her physiological gestalt. Can an infant also match *emotional* transformations it perceives in its mother to emotional transformations of its own? Extrapolating from Meltzoff's studies, as well as observations within a clinical psychoanalytic setting, I advance the following three related hypotheses.

The first hypothesis is that the infant's innate capacity for intermodal matching between the sensory, perceptual, and motor spheres may also operate between the infant's perceptual and affective spheres as well. Put another way, we can ask whether one function of human emotionality is as a type of sensory system[2] that is linked intermodally with other sensory and motor spheres to enable more accurate perception and communication of internal and external cues and potential dangers. Such pre-object states related to affect transmission normally pervade all later object relationships, both internalized as well as external. In fact, the innate capacity for displacement from one *sensory* modality to another, which characterizes intermodal matching, may serve as the body ego "template" for the later development of mental ego functions, which require the displacement from one *mental* modality to another. Intermodal matching is a sensorimotor precursor to what will later develop into the mental capacities for transformation of thought, emotion, and behavior. For example, intermodal matching may well be the pre-object protoform of the following mental functions:

1. Symbol formation and displacement, by which one representation is matched to an equivalent representation from a different modality.
2. Reaction formation and isolation, by which one affect is matched to an equivalent affect of a different modality.
3. Undoing, by which one action is matched to an equivalent action of a different modality.
4. Projection, by which a disavowed self-representation is matched to and replaced by an equivalent object representation.

---

[2]That such transmission of affect states constitutes an innate unconscious sensory modality distinguishes it from so-called telepathy or extrasensory perception. Freud (1925b) defined telepathy as "the reception of a mental process by one person from another by means *other* than sensory perception" (p. 136; emphasis added)." While the processes described in this paper might go a long way in providing an explanation for the "telepathic" processes Freud was convinced existed, I believe they are based on sensory perception, albeit of a primitive kind, that enables affects to be unconsciously transferred from one person to another.

5. Identification, by which a self-representation is matched to and altered along the lines of an equivalent object representation.
6. Projective and introjective identification, by which a disavowed self-representation in internal reality is matched to and induced in an equivalent object in external reality and vice versa.

The pre-object substrate of the representational world may therefore underlie such later-developing mental ego capacities as the principle of multiple function. Just as all sensorimotor modalities speak the same language at birth, all developing mental defenses and functions may also speak this same language, thus enabling the various parts of the personality to interrelate and enabling psychosomatic interrelation between mind and body. Disturbances of this pre-object capacity would thus have far-reaching developmental consequences, interfering with the development of the synthetic function of the ego, psychosomatic integration, and the substrate of thought and emotion.

These ideas relate to Bion's theory of thinking and to my second hypothesis. Bion (1962b) suggested that thought has two substrates: alpha- and beta-function. Alpha-function operates on the sense impressions of emotional experience, producing alpha-elements that lead to memory, symbol formation, dreaming, and verbal thought. Disturbances of alpha-function that render it inoperative lead to a state in which the sense impressions of emotional experience can no longer be transformed into symbolic thought but result, instead, in the formation of beta-elements, experienced as concrete "things-in-themselves." Bion asserted that beta-elements do not lead to dream formation (as do alpha-elements) but, rather, to projective identification and acting out. Bion (1959) further suggested that disturbances in either the infant's "inborn disposition" or in the mother's capacity to mediate the infant's distress in her reverie lead to an attack on the infant's link to the mother and thus to a developmental arrest in the infant's capacity to think and to learn from experience. What is left is a plethora of beta-particles and bizarre objects (Bion, 1957) fit only for the projective identification "of all the perceptual apparatus including the embryonic thought which forms a link between sense impressions and consciousness" (Bion, 1959, p. 107).

The relation between Meltzoff's concept of intermodal matching and Bion's concept of alpha-function is intriguing. As described by both authors, each phenomena is centrally involved in the transformation of sense impressions. Since such transformations are innate, normal, pre-objectal, and required for the link between infant and mother, both phenomena are essential for mental growth. They differ insofar as alpha-function has a more specific domain than intermodal matching. As conceptualized by their authors, alpha function operates exclusively on the sense impressions of emotion and leads to the transformation of emotional experience into symbolic thought, whereas intermodal matching yokes all sense impressions together and transforms them into other sense impressions of a different modality, while not specifically leading to the development of the semiotic function.

In order to better integrate Bion's theory of alpha-function with Meltzoff's observations of intermodal matching, I find it useful to consider the possibility of a third function. This function, which could be called "gamma-function," grows out of the infant's prestructured attachment drive and forms the normal substrate of all links that intermodally attach. Gamma function is the glue that links infant and mother, subject and object, psyche and soma, affects and sensation. Gamma-function enables the various parts of one's mind to communicate with one another and enables one to maintain the normal part-object relation with oneself described by Bion, as well as to maintain the normal cohesion of self-experience described by Kohut. Normal development in gamma-function would lead to its transformation into alpha-function, symbol formation, and the capacity for dreaming and for verbal thought. Disturbance in gamma-function would profoundly impair the infant's nascent capacity for intermodal matching and would ultimately lead to the pathological, concrete agglomeration of mental and emotional activity Bion described as a beta-particle. (In later chapters I describe how early disturbances in gamma-function and in the pre-object relatedness of infant and mother lead to two characteristic forms of pathology based on withdrawn or chaotic relatedness patterns.)

The third hypothesis is that the capacity for intermodal matching does not end in infancy with the development of symbolic mental representations but persists normally throughout life as a characteristic of primary process thought. This enables humans (perhaps like other mammalian species) to unconsciously transmit and receive affect states without speech. I call such a capacity "intermodal exchange." Intermodal exchange contributes silently to reality testing, adaptation, and species survival and persists as a form of presymbolic thought and nonverbal communication that runs parallel to that of representational thought and speech.

If I am correct in extending Meltzoff's research to suppose that humans can also match and exchange affect states intermodally, and that such capacities extend into adulthood, then it would follow that there is an isomorphism of affect elicited and affect felt. This isomorphism does not rely exclusively on either mental representations as conceptualized by Freud or on fantasy as conceptualized by Klein. For example, a parent's ability to intuit the nature of his or her infant's needs or an individual's ability to accurately read another person's mood from a facial expression, a posture, a tone of voice, or a physical gesture may predate learning and rely on a human ability to intermodally match cues from one sensory modality to a matching emotional feeling. This is not to say that the representational world does not play a significant part. In the judging of another's emotions representations are perhaps necessary but not sufficient. Because of the capacity for intermodal exchange, affects are contagious. One might speculate that the innate ability to transmit and receive affects without words may be a specific human endowment related to species survival. A patient of mine described this well when she said that, for her, the ability to vigilantly read other people's emotions played an important protective role in her development and in her relation to the world as an adult. She added: "When something deprives me of this ability it is like being deprived of one of my senses, like losing my sight or my touch."

The normal infant innately knows how to mold to its mother's moods as surely as to her touch. The infant registers these emotions in its facial expressions (Izard, 1971). Ordinary good-enough caregivers also know innately how to mold themselves to the moods and capacities of their infant. Meltzoff (1990), for example, has demonstrated that infants prefer adults who are actively imitating them. Papousek and Papousek (1979) described a range of "intuitive parenting behaviors," such as "baby talk," maintaining visual contact, exaggerated expressiveness, and speaking in a musical and high-pitched voice. These unconscious behaviors, which are in the service of initiating and maintaining social relatedness with the baby, do not have to be taught and are inhibited when brought to a parent's attention.

These observations about affect transmission may bear on Freud's conviction about the existence of telepathic phenomena, which he cited in his 1925 addendum to "The Interpretation of Dreams." Freud wrote that "thought-transference . . . comes about . . . at the moment at which an idea [which is "strongly emotionally colored"] . . . passes over from the 'primary process' to the 'secondary process' " (p. 138). Developmentally, this could refer to the infant's affect passing from its own primary processes to its mother's secondary process. A corollary of this statement is that the unconscious efforts which patient and therapist make to mold to each other's moods and needs characterize and structure the transference and countertransference.

Intermodal Matching of Affect States

In a paper on the unconscious mental activity of categorization Epstein (1992), studying adults from a neurobiological–psychoanalytic perspective, describes processes quite similar to those described by Meltzoff. Epstein observes that a fundamental quality of unconscious mentation is the organization and maintenance of associated items. Pointing to neuroanatomical and aphasia studies, Epstein notes that functional attributes of the nervous system are organized into differentiated and discrete pathways and cellular groupings. These functional groupings are associated and linked by the categorization process.

> Associative thought mechanisms are characteristic of mental life, including the infrahuman, as may be surmised by the voluminous literature on animal conditioning. An automatic associative process, occurring below awareness, has adaptive (survival) value. Upon encountering a life-threatening event in a given location, the organism finds this location is now linked to fear, so that identical or similar locations will evoke vigilance. The similar locations share an attribute and become items in the category of "dangerous places." (p. 95)

However, categorization does not rely solely on representational qualities but on prerepresentational and even physiological similarities. For example, Epstein cites studies that demonstrate that unconscious categorization can trigger epileptic seizures. Because categories have a neural substrate, Epstein postulates that, "like all neural events, category activity is subject to inhibitory–excitatory pressures with consequent potential for dysregulation" (p. 91). One wonders to what degree the categorization process described by Epstein relies on the innate intermodal matching across discrete pathways described by Meltzoff and his fellow researchers. Epstein notes that "in order for a category to become meaningful, to have survival value, it must have the capacity to become linked to an affect. An affect carries pleasurable and/or painful feeling tone. It is likely that all items in a category share an affect to some degree" (p. 96).

The mechanism allowing for the sharing of affects among discrete members of the neural categories described by Epstein might very well be that of intermodal exchange based on matching processes. In her discussion of a biological perspective on empathy Brothers (1989) suggests, as I do, that affect states can be exchanged by a process of somatic mimicry. She cites Basch (1983), who wrote:

> A given affective expression by a member of a particular species tends to recruit a similar response in other members of that species. This is done through the promotion of an unconscious, automatic, and in adults not necessarily obvious, imitation of the sender's bodily state and facial expression by the receiver. This then generates in the receiver the autonomic response associated with that bodily state and facial expression, which is to say the receiver experiences an affect identical with that of the sender. (p. 18)

Brothers also cites evidence from comparative primatological studies that supports the idea that sophisticated social communication is a hallmark of the evolution of primates. She points to studies of human and nonhuman primate infants that reveal the presence of innate and early responses to facial expression and suggest that "the phenomenon in man appears to be a product of both species evolution and individual history" (p. 17).

Let me reiterate that it is not necessary to postulate that the infant in any way initially consciously intends for its affect-driven behavior to serve as a communication to its caretakers. Affective communication is, in its most primitive state, premotivational.

However, parents discriminate between their infant's different emotional expressions and respond differently according to the nature
of the signal. The parent responds differently to a coo than to a cry.
In this way, the infant's affects signal the caretaker long before they
serve a signal function for the infant itself. This ability of the
good-enough mother to understand her infant's needs may in part
be based on the mother's utilization of her own capacities for
cross-modal matching. This would be an example of innate caretaking capacities, the adaptive use of which Kenneth King (personal
communication, 1991) refers to as "regression in the service of the
Other." The repetitive and, for the most part, reliable functioning of
the caretaker who responds adaptively to the infant's affect as a
signal may very well enable the infant to utilize its own affects for
their signal qualities from the start. In this sense, pre-object identification can be thought of as a form of emotional cross-modal
matching that enables the infant to receive or internalize its
mother's affect-regulating actions prior to the development of signal
affects, intentional signaling behavior, or even a structured representational world.

Daniel Stern (1985b) like Meltzoff, poses the question of
whether the infant's ability to match the facial expression of an adult
corresponds to a cross-modal correspondence between what the
infant sees on the adult's face and a proprioceptive configuration for
the infant's own face or whether the adult's facial expression merely
releases an innate motor program. According to Stern (1985b):

> Infants . . . appear to have an innate general capacity, which can be
> called *amodal perception,* to take information received in one sensory
> modality and somehow translate it into another sensory modality. We
> do not know how they accomplish this task. The information is prob-
> ably not experienced as belonging to any one particular sensory mode.
> More likely it transcends mode or channel and exists in some unknown
> supra-modal form. It is not, then, a simple issue of a direct translation
> across modalities. Rather, it involves an encoding into a still mysteri-
> ous amodal *representation,* which can then be recognized in any of the
> sensory modes. (p. 51; emphasis in original)

Stern goes on to demonstrate how the infant's capacity for
amodal representation contributes to the cohesion of emerging
experiences of self and other. He takes as an example the mother's
breast. The infant, as has been previously believed, does not split

up the breast as perceived by the various sensory modalities into, for example, a "seen breast," a "sucked breast," or a "touched breast." According to Stern, the "unlearned yoking" of visual and tactile sensations of the mother's breast is amodally integrated into an experience of part of another. Or, stated differently, the breast is perceived from the start as part of an Other. "The same is true for the infant's finger or fist, as seen and sucked, as well as for many other common experiences of self and other. Infants do not need repeated experience to begin to form some of the pieces of an emergent self and other. They are *predesigned* to forge certain integrations" (Stern, 1985b, p. 52; emphasis added).

Stern's point of view is similar to the one advanced here, namely, that amodal perception extends to the perception of affects. According to Stern, such perceptual capacities involve not only the infant's amodal perception of differentiated affects such as happiness or sadness but also the perception of what he calls "vitality affects." Vitality affects relate to nuances in the psychosomatic experience of affect states. Examples of vitality affects, that is, fluctuating sensuous experiences which are the currency of infant sensation, include the rush of feelings, the building up of tension, the release of tears, and the bursting of rage.

The early amodal perception of affect enables the infant to make use of its parent's efforts at affect modulation and affect regulation. In this sense, the parent's caretaking actions in support of the infant's ego functioning may be one source of Stern's "mysterious amodal representations" that enables the infant to recognize and construct for itself a bearable signal affect representation of its own previously unbearable affect state. This may be the prestage of what later develops into the infant's more differentiated relation to the parent's affect attunement and its capacity to differentiate self-representations from object-representations.

APPLICATION OF THE CONCEPT OF INTERMODAL EXCHANGE TO A THEORY OF PROJECTIVE IDENTIFICATION

The role of amodal perception and exchange of emotions between infant and mother to the development of internalized affect regulation demonstrates how the concept of projective identification can be integrated with contemporary infant developmental theory and research. One of the primary sources of controversy about the concept of projective identification is a lack of clarity about the means by which aspects of the self-representation are thought to be projected *into* another individual and then, after being modified by that individual, subsequently reinternalized. While the concept of projective identification is very useful clinically, some of the literature about it has an unfortunately concrete tone, as though affects and disavowed aspects of the self were flying about the room entering and controlling people.

The conundrum about how projective identification actually operates has been viewed by most authors from two disparate points of view. The first point of view understands projective identification concretely as involving an actual installation of one's affects into the interior of another individual and the subsequent reinternalization of the now modified affects from the interior of the object back to the interior of the self (Bion, 1959; Grotstein, 1985; Malin and Grotstein, 1966). The second point of view maintains that the self and its objects are first and foremost individuals and that projective identification can only be thought of as a *fantasy* of projection into the object, with subsequent actualizing behaviors based on this fantasy (Ogden, 1979, 1982; Sandler, 1987a).

By emphasizing the separateness of the individuals involved in the process of projective identification the second point of view tends to view infant–mother interactions and archaic mental processes through the lens of differentiated adult mental processes. Defining projective identification as a fantasy rather than as a concrete exchange moves the concept forward developmentally to a time following the baby's acquisition of symbolic mental processes. If Winnicott was right in declaring that the baby cannot properly be considered as separate from the environmental provision of its mother, then we clearly need a different way of conceptualizing the emotion-laden interchanges between infant and mother that occur in a subjectively undifferentiated matrix. We also need a way to understand the archaic emotional communications by which one individual is able uncannily to introduce effects of his or her own feelings into another individual.[3]

---

[3]Sandler (1976) makes clear that what one who has "received" a projective identification experiences is not, in fact, a replica of what has been externalized but a compromise between what the other individual has projected and one's own thoughts and feelings.

This returns us to the dilemma posed by psychoanalytic theory of having to choose between (1) a baby who is capable of somehow installing its affects directly into its mother and searching for her affects to be installed into itself but who is not yet possessed of the differentiated symbolic mental representations of self and object necessary for such transactions to occur and (2) a baby who possesses a representational world enabling it to differentiate itself from its mother enough to be capable of projective identification but who is too separate to be engaging in concrete presymbolic merged transactions with her.

Further, and most important, neither of these points of view specifies the means by which projective identification takes place. The first, or merged, view argues for a concept of concrete projection of affects into the mother's interior but does not describe how such an action can take place. The second view, by describing projective identification in postdifferentiated terms, so subordinates the concept to higher-level processes of identification and projection that the value of a concept of direct emotional transfer is lost.

The view that emerges from the perspective of pre-object relatedness is of a neonate who *does* possess a rudimentary representational capacity, although a presymbolic one not previously considered by psychoanalysts or cognitive psychologists as being truly representational. Although psychoanalytic research has tended to equate a representational capacity with the semiotic function of symbolic thought, Meltzoff and his colleagues have demonstrated the existence in infants of a capacity for supramodal representation based upon an inborn capacity for intermodal exchange between sensory modalities. It is possible to surmise that *intermodal exchange is the means by which affects are concretely transferred between infant and mother and, later, between adults.* By considering projective identification as a form of *intermodal exchange* it is possible to account theoretically for the concrete transfer of affects and sensations between two individuals—even when one of the individuals is an infant who is months away from developing a representational world based on mental images and symbolic thought.

In fact, in light of what is emerging from infant research, psychoanalysis may be in need of a broader definition of the concept of the representational world, that is, a revision that would not limit the definition of a representation to a purely mental image. Laplanche and Pontalis (1973), for example, point out that a feeling or a behavior is just as likely to be the concrete expression of a representation as is a mental image. Pre-objectal experiences based on intermodal exchange of affect states can thus be thought of as a component of the representational world, albeit not in the form of symbolic ideational thought.

In normal development such intermodal exchanges are the means by which an infant elicits from its caregivers and subsequently internalizes adaptive responses based upon its parent's affective attunement. These adaptive responses become experienced as part of the core self. While the increasingly internalized ability to elicit adaptive responses lays the groundwork for later development of secondarily autonomous ego functions related to affect regulation and affect recognition, ego defenses, reality sense, self-caring abilities, insight, and empathy, this pre-object dimension of human experiencing and human relating is related more to primary process, primary autonomy, and primary identification. Bollas (1989) aptly calls these central aspects of the self—that is, the infant's sense of a core self and ability to recognize and adapt to its own needs—the "idiom" of the person. Hartmann (1948, 1950a, b, 1953, 1955, 1964) and other ego psychologists demonstrated that these capacities are intimately connected in part with innate biological and genetic sources, and Winnicott (1949, 1958a, 1965, 1971b, 1989) called attention to the part played by the internalization of environmental effects. The interaction of these influences is complex, but a consensus supports the conclusion that disturbance of the primary attachment figures' adaptive responses to the infant's biological and ego needs produces disturbances in the development of the infant's signaling behavior and impairment of the infant's capacities to internalize and regulate its own disturbed affect states.

CHAPTER FIVE

Intermodal Exchange and the Psychoanalytic Situation

I N WHAT WAY do primordial experiences normally endure into adulthood and make their presence felt in the psychoanalytic situation? In our offices physical touch, for example, is excluded, but we can feel touched by our patients' emotions and they can feel touched by our empathy. Might intermodal exchange of affect states be a pre-object function of the primary process? According to Dorpat (1991), the secondary process involves itself with conscious and rational cognition whereas the primary process unconsciously attends to affective, object-relational information. The two are constantly woven together in all mental activity. Such a way of thinking about the pre-object aspects of the unconscious might enable us to encompass in our theories what previously had been thought to be ineffable or uncanny in the psychoanalytic situation.

INTUITION AND INTERMODAL EXCHANGE

I have noticed over the years that I am often able to sense when a patient has had a dream, often before the patient has remembered it. I do not fully know how I am able to do this, but from informal conversations with other analysts and psychotherapists I have concluded that this ability is not at all uncommon. I don't understand the cognitive steps I take to reach this knowledge but I am not usually mistaken. I have assumed that the ability to intuit my patient's inner state arises out of what Sandler (1976) has called the analyst's "role-responsiveness," that is, "the capacity to allow all sorts of thoughts, day-dreams and associations to enter the analyst's consciousness while he is at the same time listening to and observing the patient" (p. 44).

If I were to generalize my own personal experience of role-responsiveness, I would describe something like this: A patient is talking about his life, perhaps with some sense of urgency or conflict, although the source of the conflict is unclear. I listen to the patient's associations, but they seem to suggest no deeper meaning to me. I have a frustrating sense that there is nothing to analyze, while at the same time I am convinced that something important is occurring. Similarly, the nature of the patient's mood seems unclear and I find myself unable to feel attuned emotionally to the patient. Before too long the thought occurs to me, "If the patient had had a dream last night, this might all be clearer." Sometimes at this point I ask the patient directly if he has recently had a dream. Very often the patient has a startled reaction and says something like, "How did you know? I had a dream last night but had forgotten about it until just now." The session usually then proceeds more typically, with analysis of the dream resolving most further questions about the nature of that day's unconscious conflict. However, concerned that such questions interrupt the spontaneous process of an analysis, I now tend to refrain from asking directly for dreams. I have since persuaded myself that "fishing" for dreams, as Winnicott used to call the practice, is usually unnecessary, and I have noticed that shortly after I begin to wonder—silently—whether the patient has dreamed, often the person will pause momentarily and say, "I just remembered; I had a dream last night."

Freud described the analyst's receptivity to the patient's unconscious and how, over time, the analyst's unconscious or preconscious mental processes become matched to those of the patient. Yet the way this happens has remained unknown. In my view, an understanding of intermodal matching of affect states as an innate response subserving the developmental, adaptive, and survival interests of the infant as well as the species provides a way to better understand such seemingly mysterious processes. The intermodal exchange of affect states would explain how newborns are able to communicate their needs to their caregivers prior to the development of the functional ego capacities required to mentally represent those needs as signal affects. Further, the concept of intermodal exchange makes more understandable the means by which infants are able to internalize the affect states of their mothers. An innate capacity for intermodal "knowledge" based on the matching of affect states would explain why an infant cries irritably and holds its body in rigid extension when held anxiously by its mother but molds its body to its mother's body and feels soothed when held reassuringly. Similarly, adult processes of intermodal matching might account for the way in which a mother often discovers herself awakening in the middle of the night just before her baby has begun to cry. Despite being asleep, a mother remains attuned to minute clues from the adjacent room and responds to the implications of small sounds that others might not notice—a shift in respiration, a movement, perhaps the absence of a sound that signifies sleep.[1]

But how should we describe what is happening in this process? Does the sleeping mother mentally represent the imminent awakening of her child as much as she senses it? Does the sleeping mother comprehend the imminent awakening of her infant, or does she apprehend it? If we compare the nursing situation to the psychoanalytic situation, to the analyst who has a hunch that the patient has dreamed even though he or she has not yet been told of the dream, might we say that the analyst has "awakened" from the patient's dream just before the patient has? And does the analyst in such an instance know the patient's unconscious, or does he or she feel it? What wordless sounds or actions has the patient made to communicate the presence of a dream? Certainly, a more comprehensive

---

[1]Perhaps, too, the baby awakens and cries shortly after its mother awakens, each one matched to the sounds the other makes in the night. James McKenna (Manson, 1993), an anthropologist at Pomona College, has begun an interesting study, funded by the National Institutes of Health, of the connection between infant isolation and crib death, known as sudden infant death syndrome (SIDS). Statistics indicate that the incidence of SIDS in the United States, Britain, Canada, Australia, and New Zealand, societies in which infants and mothers generally sleep apart, is five times as high as in Hong Kong, Pakistan, Japan, and Bangladesh, societies in which infants and mothers customarily share the same bed for the baby's first year. Pilot tests seems to indicate that when mothers and infants sleep together, the infant's breathing patterns, heart rates, and sleep stages follow their mothers'. McKenna notes that solitary infant sleep has only become the norm in Western civilization in the last 200 years, since the Industrial Revolution. He hypothesizes that this trend was prompted by society's demand for staunch individualism and by myths and fears that babies who shared their mother's bed will grow up to be overly dependent.

notion of the processes involved is gained by taking into account the intermodal exchanges and other pre-representational experiences that link the emotionality of the mother and infant, the analyst and patient.

On occasion mothers have brought their babies to their psychoanalytic sessions. This has given me the opportunity to observe the effect of the mother's psychoanalysis *upon her infant*. It will come as no surprise that this is not a scientifically controlled study, but there is enough similarity between observations that I feel there is some use in repeating them here. A frequent observation involves the mother who enters the analytic office tense and anxious with a baby who is fretting, fussing, and irritable. The mother believes she is tense because her baby won't calm down and let her participate fully in her session. Her mothering of the infant is often perfunctory and unempathic, and her movements are jerky. As the session proceeds, the mother's free associations generally reveal the presence of some unconscious conflict, which I attempt to address in the usual psychoanalytic manner by way of a verbal interpretation. Here is what I often notice: If the interpretation of the mother's conflict is apt, *her baby calms down*. In part this can be explained by the fact that the mother becomes more attuned to and accepting of her baby's feelings as she becomes more aware of and accepting of her own feelings. The mother's physical caretaking abilities noticeably improve, and her movements with the infant become better synchronized with the baby's movements—more fluid, less jerky. All of this can be described in plain language by saying that the mother relaxes after the correct interpretation is made. From the perspective of her capacity for object relatedness, this temporarily improved affect regulation enables the patient to mother more effectively (Anderson, 1995). From the perspective of her capacity for pre-object relatedness, the mother's newfound calmness is transmitted directly to her infant via an intermodal exchange, which enables the baby to be calmer or to fall asleep. I believe that this transmission of relief is direct and does not rely on an intervening symbolic representation.

In speaking of prerepresentational states I should perhaps clarify my terminology and stress that I do not mean nonrepresentational but something more akin to a precursor of a mental image, which is itself a precursor of a mental representation. I refer to the concept of representation in the psychoanalytic sense, that is, as a stable configuration of linked, emotionally charged mental images. Sandler and Rosenblatt (1962) describe a representation as having

> a more or less enduring existence as an organization or schema which is constructed out of a multitude of impressions. A child experiences many images of his mother—mother feeding, mother talking, mother sitting down, mother standing up, mother preparing food, etc.—and on the basis of these gradually creates a mother representation which encompasses a whole range of mother images, all of which bear the label "mother." (p. 133)

In the context of this way of thinking about the representational world, pre-object experiences signify the beginnings of what will later be the capacity to think of one's self in relation to the enduring construct of an independent other (i.e., an object relationship). However, pre-object experiences do not yet mentally represent an object relationship. Recourse to a metaphor might be helpful in explaining further what I mean. Television sets take a few seconds to warm up before a picture or sound appears. Pre-object states might at first be no more representational than the small, bright dot in the center of the television screen that has just been turned on. At first the observer cannot be certain whether the center of light will grow into the full-blown pictures and sounds of "Masterpiece Theatre" or "The Simpsons." The dot, while not representing the full array of audio and video signals, at least indicates that the set is on and that the signal is beginning to be received and projected onto the screen. While the transmission and reception of the human emotional signal is "instant-on," the baby's representational world has to warm up a bit before pictures, words, and meanings appear.

There is a similar distinction to be drawn when considering the inborn existence of a capacity for supramodal representations. Such supramodal capabilities are still prerepresentational in the psychoanalytic sense, because they are not yet encompassed within an imagined representational world of related and differentiated images of self and object. However, supramodal representations serve as the sensorimotor *precursors* for the later development of fully mental representation. This innate capacity for supramodality is a manifestation of a gamma-function that links the infant's sensory and mental capacities to the physical support and emotional nurture it receives from its caregivers. Such yoking of soma, psyche, and environmental support makes emotional development possible. One paradox of this development is that the baby's individuation grows out of a symbiotic matrix of intermodal equivalence. This intermodal equivalence between the sensory and affective modalities of the infant and mother makes the neonate's capacity for mental representation possible while not, in itself, being representable to the infant. Because of this distinction, clinical experiences based on pre-object modes of communication are different in quality and type from experiences based on more advanced forms of unconscious communication that have developed after the establishment of a capacity for internalized object relations.

SYMBOLIC AND PRESYMBOLIC COMMUNICATION

Two similar situations, occurring within the same month in my practice, illustrate some of the differences between pre-object modes of communication and advanced forms of unconscious communication.

> A young father in psychotherapy was describing what felt to him like a conflict of loyalties toward his wife and his son. He related this to his conviction that in the past he had been indirectly culpable in the deaths of two family members. He thought this oppressive sense of responsibility was irrational, yet he still could not shake it. Now he felt the pressing need to undo the earlier losses by vigilantly overprotecting his son in order to prevent any harm from befalling him.
>
> Preliminary to an effort to further analyze the unconscious sources of his conflict, I tried to summarize his description of how he felt. I said, "It sounds as though you feel a bit like a catcher in the rye, catching all the children as they come through the rye field and before they fall over the edge of a cliff."
>
> The man looked startled and immediately said, "That's just what I dreamed last night! In the dream I was holding my son in my arms and I came to the edge of a cliff. I clutched him to me to prevent his falling over the edge."

The next example is harder to describe and so requires more explanation:

> The patient was in her last trimester of pregnancy with her third child. During the sessions preceding the one to be described the woman had felt overwhelmed by all the responsibilities she felt she had to meet. Although she had developed a medical complication that potentially involved the need for rapid hospitalization for the induction of labor, her husband was about to leave town on a business trip. The patient reported the information about her husband's impending absence blandly and almost as an afterthought. Struck by her seeming disinterest, I commented on it. She became aware of dreading her husband's absence and began to cry, admitting that she felt she could not convey to him how much she wanted him not to leave her. In addition, she felt she could not depend on her mother for help in his absence.
>
> At the next session, two days later, the woman looked cheerful. However, in curious contrast to her mood, she immediately reported that she had suffered a medical emergency shortly after the last session. While the emergency turned out to be controllable with medication, she had required overnight hospitalization and multiple medical tests and interventions.
>
> However, despite the fact that the patient was telling me about her emergency, I found myself becoming drowsy. I found it curious that my response was so out of keeping with the content of what the patient was saying to me, yet I continued to become sleepier and sleepier. For some reason, I felt more alert when I heard the patient say that as a result of the medical emergency her husband had decided on his own to cancel his business trip and her mother-in-law had decided to fly in to help her. Summarizing what she seemed to be telling me, I said, "So despite the emergency, something good seemed to come out of it." Now I suddenly felt wide awake. The patient immediately responded, "Yes, and you know what? I was so relieved that I got the first good night's sleep last night that I have had in weeks!" I had not previously known that the patient had been having trouble sleeping.

Now, both clinical experiences strike me as superficially similar in the sense that I was able somehow to intuit an inner state of the patient without having been told about it directly. In the first case I unwittingly described a patient's manifest dream before he told me about it. In the second case I felt sleepy just before a patient told me about her good night's sleep. Yet in a deeper sense the experiences also strike me as dissimilar. In my view, the first is an example of a communication conveyed by unconscious verbal associations and symbolic thought while the second example is related to a form of affect transmission between patient and analyst.

Let me begin with the first example of the felicitous use of the "catcher in the rye" metaphor. Months of preceding sessions, countless derivative verbal communications, and many previously reported dreams had, by accretion, already formed in me a mental representation of the patient as defined by his prevailing conflict. I had already formulated private hypotheses concerning the unconscious derivatives of that conflict, which I had not yet spoken of to the patient. To take just one example, I wondered to what extent his conscious irrational feeling of responsibility was unconsciously rational in the sense that he had, prior to these family members' deaths, actually wished to be rid of them. To the patient's horror, the subsequent deaths were like a wish come true. Consequently, his resentment and anger now terrified him, and he thought of himself as a killer. He had to stand guard against himself, constantly repressing, undoing, and guiltily expiating his angry wishes.

Although the metaphor of the catcher in the rye seemed to come to me intuitively as I spoke, I can, in retrospect, operationalize the preconscious steps I took to reach this formulation. I knew that any direct interpretation of the patient's destructive fantasies would certainly bring on a wave of guilt and self-recrimination. Therefore, preliminary to any exploration of what to him was his dangerous aggression I thought it best to bring to his attention the reality of his protective and reparative motives, that is, to analyze his defense before his impulse (A. Freud, 1936). I also was motivated by my wish to say something to him that conveyed my sense of empathy for the burden his unconscious conflict placed upon him.

But how had I arrived at the precise "catcher in the rye" metaphor, which so closely mirrored the patient's dream? First, the patient had already described the sense that he was standing guard over his son, the preposition *over* signifying a spatial relationship in which he was above his child. I knew from previous sessions that the family member whose death he felt most guilty about had died in a fall. In this context the metaphor of his standing guard over his child to prevent him from falling to his death came to me naturally. However, the steps I just described were out of my conscious awareness; at the time my comment just seemed like the appropriate thing to say. When the patient responded by telling me the dream he had had the night before, the dream confirmed the validity of my suppositions concerning the nature of the patient's unconscious conflict and allowed us to explore the extent to which he feared the occasions of his own normal and expectable frustration and anger with his son.

Reassured of the reality of his reparation, the patient was able in subsequent sessions to acknowledge his hateful wishes toward his son and the family members who had died. He also became more aware of his sense of shame, guilt, and remorse over what felt to him to be the omnipotence of his destructiveness. For example, he began to realize that he had been feeling resentful and frightened because he sensed that his son was beginning to grow away from him, even though he knew that this was developmentally normal and desirable. Partly because of this resentment and fear, he had been planning to father another child. Thus, the dream of clutching his son to prevent his falling over the cliff represented not only his wish to keep his son from growing up and separating from him but also a reaction formation against his wish to "drop" this child by having another one. There had been, of course, significant past betrayals, losses, and rejections out of which the patient's present vulnerability grew. These emotions and the relationships to which they were linked were all mentally represented in his inner world, although they were repressed. He had verbally communicated these emotions to me, and I had formed a mental representation of the patient, which I preconsciously utilized in order to formulate my interpretation.

I think the second clinical example, in which I began to feel sleepy, is better described as a form of intermodal exchange. Such affect transmission serves as a substrate of but predates verbal speech, symbolic thought, mental representation, and internalized affect regulation. The capacity for protorepresentational communication is apparently already present at birth and would certainly seem to have a high value for species survival. This is not to say that verbal representation and secondary process thought had no role in this interaction. Certainly, the patient may have felt that I, like her husband and mother, was abandoning her, since our next appointment was not for another two days and since I had not helped her to give voice to her feelings about my absence in the preceding session. But perhaps, simultaneously, my sleepy response was an example of my attunement to the content of her emotional state rather than to the content of her speech. I was hearing and responding more to the happiness and relief in her tone of voice than to her description of the averted catastrophe. Because of her tone of voice and physical relaxation on the couch I intuitively understood that her story was going to have a happy ending, so I could relax and grow sleepy, as she had.

I was not able to represent these realizations to the patient, as was possible in the example of my "catcher in the rye" statement. Rather, the effect on me was psychosomatic. In retrospect, I think I can translate what happened into representational terms: My sleepiness mirrored the patient's experience of the physical or emotional unavailability of those she most depended on as well as her experience of relief and relaxation. Yet I would argue that had this sense of abandonment and relief been conveyed representationally at the time, this subsequent step of translation would not have been necessary. As it was, I responded to the patient's intermodal transmission of sleepiness, concretely beginning to relinquish the central ego function of consciousness in a kind of somatic mimicry of her, although she had said or implied nothing about her good night's sleep. Furthermore, I also seemed to mimic her intermodal communication of alert repose, by "waking up" to make my comment that something good seemed to come out of the emergency.

PSYCHOANALYTIC PROCESS
AND PRIMARY RELATEDNESS

Eugenio Gaddini (1992) links intermodal exchanges between patient and analyst to the deepest nonverbal aspects of the state of primary relatedness:

> In this process the contribution of the environment (mother, breast) is fundamental, but what is most important is that this *precedes the*

instinctual relationship with the object. . . . *Where the process of "creation of the self"* (Winnicott) is somehow disturbed, the result is a pathology of the self which will interfere more or less severely with the development of the instinctual relationship and hence with the identificatory processes and the formation of the subject's own identity. In such cases, the analytical relationship must be able to operate on very deep levels, remote from language, and barely if at all instinctual. Verbal interpretation at instinctual levels may in these cases have no meaning, whereas silence and participation may assume an important therapeutic function. (p. 100; emphasis in original)

Gaddini cites Winnicott, who wrote the following in *Playing and Reality*:

It is only in recent years that I have become able to wait and wait for the natural evolution of the transference arising out of the patient's growing trust in the psychoanalytic technique and setting, and to avoid breaking up this natural process by making interpretations. It appalls me to think of how much deep change I have prevented or delayed in patients in a certain classification category by my personal need to interpret. (cited in Gaddini, 1992, p. 100)

Gaddini (1992) asserts that in the analysis of primitive aspects of the transference what matters most is not the transference interpretation of the patient's instinctual relationship to the analyst but "the analyst's ability to be 'involvable' in the relationship at the level required by the patient. Responding in the appropriate ways to the relationship of magical contact in which the patient puts himself means extending the therapy to the needs of a self that were not sufficiently met at the relevant time" (p. 101).

Meeting these inchoate needs as they emerge in states of deep regression in the psychoanalytic transference can lead to a fundamental repair of early traumatic states, but this work is often horrifying for the patient and analyst because it often approximates disintegration and can often be confused with deterioration (Casement, 1982; Kinston and Cohen, 1986; Kumin, 1985–1986, 1986; Winnicott, 1974).

An example of this comes from the analysis of a man who was adopted in infancy and was told of his adoption when he was three. After six years of analysis, during which he had repeatedly kept his emotional distance from any ideas I had that the adoption had been important to him, he set a termination date some months in the future.

Shortly after setting the termination date, he dreamed that he was in a twin-propeller airplane in the act of taking off. The runway was bumpy and seemed to be too short. He was unsure whether or not to abort the takeoff. If he attempted to fly and the runway was indeed not long enough, a disastrous crash would ensue.

The dream seemed to indicate that the help the patient had received in the tumultuous ("bumpy") analysis—the twin-motor aircraft represented the holding environment and the selfobject transference—was enabling him to "fly" for the first time in his life, that is, to separate and individuate, to leave his depression behind, to feel mature and adult, to even consider leaving the analysis and me. But he could not differentiate genuinely flying on his own from manic flight. He was terrified about the consequences of termination, afraid he would suffer a depressive "crash," because he felt the analysis had not been long enough to help him resolve something crucial.

Shortly afterward the patient was told by doctors that he suffered from a congenital spinal condition in his neck that might worsen one day and eventually lead to paralysis. He anguished about his fate incessantly, was in terror that he would lose bowel and bladder control, and suffered constant cervical neck pain. He decided against leaving analysis until he came to better terms with his illness.

He dreamed that he was having surgery but wasn't totally asleep. He was in the middle of a painful situation that he would have to experience. But he was too asleep to cry out for help. After the surgery, the surgeon told him that because she could get no closer than three centimeters to the lesion, he was going to have to live with the problem.

While the dream related to the patient real concerns about the surgery he might need, it related to the emergence of painful feelings about his adoption as well. My conjecture was that the surgery in the dream symbolized the severing of his attachment to his birth mother. While he was aware of the excruciating pain of the loss, it was too early for him to be conscious enough to signal his distress. When he was told of the adoption by his parents at the age of three, it was too late to do anything to change the loss; he just had to learn to live with it. Further, the dream indicated that he understood increasingly that he would have to experience this early pain in the "surgery" of the analysis and that the anesthesia of his denial was preventing him from recognizing that he desperately wanted my help and was preventing me from getting close enough to assist him. In a way, he was always creating his own losses because he distanced himself from those who could help him. This was represented in the dream by his "sleep" and by the surgeon who couldn't get close to the lesion. I also wondered to myself if he felt hopeless because he doubted whether all the talking in the world could ever get close enough to reach his painful preverbal experiences.

Over a period of months I continued to assist the patient in working through the source of his panic. I continued to make occasional comments based on my conjecture that his terror was related not only to the reality of his threatened paralysis but also to the reliving of his maternal loss in infancy. To him, the potential compression of his spinal cord and loss of connection to his body was unconsciously indistinguishable from the severing of his attachment to his biological mother and thus the annihilation of his self. Ending the analysis and the attachment to me was perceived as a similar catastrophic loss. The patient was not certain he could function on his own but hated his attachment to me and others. His hatred of himself made his attachments seem humiliating to him, like a dependence that rendered him a helpless, incontinent baby.

While the patient consciously rejected these interpretations, his anxiety steadily decreased and he no longer brooded incessantly about his physical condition. In one session I commented on the relation between the real threat of paralysis and the way he eradicated awareness of his emotions because he feared emotions would lead to paralyzing dependence on others. At the next session he reported this dream:

He encountered his biological mother for the first time (he had been told that she was, in fact, dead). Her back was turned to him, and an infant was tied to her. She turned slowly toward the

patient, and he viewed her face for the first time. When she saw
him for the first time, she was overcome with emotion.

In the dream his mother seemed to be the one who was experiencing strong feelings; the patient himself was unemotional about the encounter. He confirmed this observation by talking about the dream unemotionally and without much insight. I asked where the baby was attached to his mother's body. He said, without interest, "On her back." I asked where on her back. Again, without interest, he responded, "Somewhere up high, around her shoulders." "On her neck?" I asked. He burst out with rueful laughter and said, "Right!" He was then flooded with emotion.

In this dream the patient seemed to indicate that he now felt that a state of primary relatedness had been reestablished in the analysis; he equated the primary attachment to his self via his spinal cord to the primary attachment to his mother by the umbilical cord. This capacity for primary relatedness was being gradually repaired through the actual environmental mediation of the analysis. To be sure, deep experiences of early deprivation or trauma were still a significant aspect of the transference, but they were mentally represented and symbolized with increasing frequency, albeit in primitive forms, and were becoming increasingly amenable to verbal interpretation.

Assisted by the increasing awareness of his feelings about his adoption, the patient realized that he had been denying his belief that his biological mother might still be alive; an unconscious hope made manifest in this dream. He launched a search for her and eventually succeeded in finding her, as well as siblings he had not known existed. While not without conflict, the discovery was a deep relief to him and brought him a sense of wholeness and belonging that had before seemed unattainable.

COMMUNICATION TO THE BODY

Hidden meanings in verbally communicated speech, composed primarily of symbolically encoded messages, can be intuited, but the meanings of pre-object communications are generally perceived physically. For example, a patient in the first few months of analysis asked, "Do I make you anxious?" At that instant I realized for the first time that my finger was in my mouth and I was biting my nail. "Well," she added, "so anxious that you can't function as an analyst anymore?" I said something then that she found useful, and she went on to recall some early memories about difficulties in her relationship with her mother.

Pre-object communication is primarily sensorimotor in nature. It is usually sensed by the body of the analyst rather than by his or her mind. Perhaps, following Epstein (1992), one would say that primitive communications are "categorized" rather than understood. Pre-object meaning is concrete and is represented intermodally rather than symbolically. Very often, preverbal communication can literally be sensed as a gut feeling.

This quality of pre-object communication is exemplified by a female patient who after a year of analysis was in a transitory state of "erotic horror" (Kumin, 1985–1986, 1986) concerning her intensely sexualized feelings about me. One day she said with great apprehension and shame that she wanted very badly to get off the couch and come over to me. I said that she must have something specific in mind that she wanted to do with me. She said she wanted to come over to my chair and make love to me while straddling me with her legs locked tightly around me. My response to this fantasy surprised me: Rather than responding with neutrality or even excitement, I had an almost visceral reaction of entrapment. On the basis of this physical sensation and of what I knew of the woman's panic about separation and loss, I replied, "I certainly wouldn't be able to go anywhere *then*." She laughed and relaxed. "No," she said, "you'd look pretty silly at the end of the session when you went to leave and you walked into the hall with me still wrapped around your waist!" I pointed out that at the end of the session it was *she* who left, not I. She immediately became sad and remembered her uncle, one of the few adults who paid any attention to her. During her childhood he played with her affectionately whenever he visited her family. When the time came for him to leave, she would respond with panic and would throw herself onto his leg, wrapping her arms and legs around him. He would often walk to the front door dragging her along still wrapped to his leg.

Following the recovery of this memory the woman's intensely erotized transference rapidly waned, and she became calmer in her feelings about me and the analysis. The point I want to emphasize in this example is the way I was able to represent for myself an early ego state of the patient's. I did this not so much on the basis of what the patient was saying, which was manifestly sexual and seductive, but mostly on the basis of an unpleasant physical sensation induced in me by what she was feeling as the almost unbearable pressure of her own desire, desperateness, clinging, and imminent erotic horror. This panic related to the traumatic series of losses suffered by this patient during virtually every developmental phase from infancy on.

I learned more about these losses later in the analysis. I noticed that my patient was taking copious quantities of Kleenex throughout each session, whether or not she was crying, and that she usually took more "for the road" at the end of the session. One day she was bemoaning her fate in being flat-chested (she had complained on several previous occasions that she had "absolutely nothing on top"). I heard this statement not only as related to her actual body but also as referring to an inner emptiness related to deprivation in her experience of her relationship with her mother (Kumin, 1978a; 1989). I said that I wondered if she felt she had taken into herself the deprivation of her relationship with her mother as an empty, flattened, "nothing" breast, which now made her feel that she had to care entirely for herself because she could depend on no one, including me. I wondered if she perhaps consoled herself by insatiably taking more and more of my tissues as though desperately nursing at an empty breast, as though my tissues were all she could let herself count on me for.

She told me that her mother had not breast-fed her because shortly after giving birth she had suffered a severe depression that necessitated months of hospitalization. Her grandmother had moved into her home and raised her until her mother resumed her care a year later. When her mother returned home, her grandmother then moved out. In effect, my patient had lost her two primary caregivers in her first year of life. After she told me about the loss of her mother and her breast, she suddenly remembered a dream from the night before.

> *In the dream it was night. She was lost, she was alone, and she was desperately hungry. She was endlessly searching for a place where she could get something to eat.*

Over the next two weeks the woman went through a planned series of medical tests to determine the cause of some physical symptoms that were worrying her. While she knew the illness was not fatal, she was nevertheless agitated and terribly worried. She could not fathom the source of her panic. She then described having watched television coverage of the Olympics and having heard the story of Oksana Baiul, the 16-year-old Russian figure skater who had lost her father in infancy, her mother at age 12, and her foster parent/coach at 13. The skater was an orphan. I said that worry and concern were certainly justified by the unknown source of her illness but that the source of her *panic* was the feeling that she was also an orphan of a sort. And now she was sick and perhaps feeling she could no longer depend on herself or anyone else, even me. The patient agreed in a perfunctory way but then said she remembered a dream from the night before.

> *In the dream she was at her mother's house. She was outside, unearthing what appeared to be a dead plant from the ground. To her profound relief she discovered that the plant was not dead after all, that there were a few buds on its limbs that might sprout new growth.*

"And this part is really weird," she said. "As I brushed the dirt off them, the buds looked like breasts, like nipples." The patient was telling me indirectly that I had been wrong in thinking that she felt she could not depend on anyone and that, in fact, the analysis was enabling her to bring back to life a sense of hope in the future and a belief in the adequacy of her very early sensuous relationship to her mother, as recreated in the transference (Wrye and Welles, 1989, 1994).

While this example also concerns an early infantile state, it differs in kind and quality from the example of transmitted sleepiness mentioned earlier in this chapter. Here the patient is talking about the infantile state, her associations contain analyzable symbolic derivatives of that state, and she is able to dream about it. This demonstrates the beginning of her symbolic capacity to tolerate the state enough to mentally represent it. From my side, I was able to listen to the patient's associations in a state of relative emotional neutrality, decipher her unconscious meaning, and formulate reasonably accurate verbal interpretations about her latent meaning. In contrast, the pre-object communication of the earlier example, where I very nearly fell asleep, was primarily sensorimotor in nature. Pre-object relatedness is not mentally symbolized as much as it is concretely embodied.

Because primitive representation crosses sensory modalities, a gesture or a smell can arouse desire, a facial expression can trigger panic, a tone of voice can evoke deep calm, a posture can stir suspicion, a violin sonata can bring tears of regret, and the crashing of waves on a beach or the drumming of rain on a roof can summon sleep. One might argue that such physical responses are linked to affectively charged memories and thus are symbolically encoded and unconsciously deciphered. Yet I would suggest that at least some of these experiences in adulthood progress directly from one modality to another without the intermediary of memory, thought, or symbolic representation. The sound of fingernails scraping across a blackboard needs no intervening association or memory in order to evoke the shiver that immediately runs down one's spine. It is a pure intermodal response: A sound prompts a chill without an intervening thought.

Meltzoff's demonstration of the presence at birth of a kind of intermodal representation suggests a theoretically plausible modification of an aspect of Melanie Klein's hypothesis regarding the presence of very early projective and introjective mechanisms. Klein's specific scenarios of paranoid-schizoid and depressive positions have often been criticized because of the implausibility of such sophisticated representational capacities being available to infants. However, the discovery of protorepresentational capacities present at birth in the form of innate intermodal translation lends credence to the idea that emotionally charged exchanges between infant and mother are possible, based on the empathic fit of the dyad, from birth on. One may even wonder whether intermodal exchanges between fetus and mother operate prior to birth, as recent research seems to suggest (Piontelli, 1992). If so, we may surmise that one of the baby's earliest signals is a kick and that one of the mother's earliest responses is a change in heartbeat or respiratory rhythm.

Intermodal exchange is central in the creation of art, and one application of the concept of intermodal communication may be the study of its place in the creative process. In an attempt to describe the way a writer uses metaphor, John Husband, a poet and college English teacher of mine, explained that a literal description of a mood does not in fact convey the mood effectively to a reader. A mood must be evoked rather than described. The way he put it was, "One bat will do for hell." Now, one might say that this describes the function of symbolic, rather than pre-object, images as signifiers. I would claim that while the bat might symbolically represent hell, the sense of unease evoked by the implication of evil derives from intermodal links from the symbolic and mental sphere of metaphor and memory to the bodily sphere of affect. Perhaps a better example might be abstract expressionism, where a protorepresentational gestalt emerging from the canvas's color, gesture, texture, and shape can evoke deep and complex moods and memories. Some forms of humor might serve as another example. I once made an absurd rejoinder to a friend's comment. He laughed long and hard, then said, "I don't get it." I had also thought my remark was funny, although *I didn't understand what I had meant, either*! I don't remember the joke now; anyway, I am certain that even if I could repeat it here, it would not seem amusing at all. You had to be there, as they say. You had to be there because only then, I believe, would all the complex gestural, affective, and bodily intermodal signifiers be present to make the joke seem funny despite its verbal content, which was, judging by all secondary process standards, obscure at best. This is the essence of pre-object communication. *You have to be there to "get it."* Because its function is to precipitate a new sensation in another rather than to signify or approximate a past mental event, the pre-object state can only exist in the sensorimotor here-and-now of a relational field.

This may account for the observation that psychoanalytic case reports often seem flat and unconvincing: The verbal description cannot adequately convey the pre-object dimension shared by patient and analyst. Verbal transactions can be repeated, transcribed, described, symbolized, abstracted, and represented. This is because words are a form of internalized object, and internalized objects evoke mental representations. The pre-object state, by contrast, evokes concrete bodily experiences encoded as affects. Unlike verbal communication, preverbal communication is not portable. Pre-object communication cannot be repeated since it exists concretely in real time between individuals who are communicating in this way.

CHAPTER SIX

Fields of Identity

ARLY IN LIFE most people develop an internal sense of the
permanence of their loved ones as well as a cohesive and
enduring experience of themselves as individuals. These experiences of the self and its loved objects become elaborated in a
subjective representational world. This developmental milestone
occurs as the amodal pre-object dimension of early subjective experience begins to consolidate into the more stable configurations of
the mentally represented internal world of differentiated self and
objects. The failure to adequately differentiate self- from object
representations is a sign of psychopathology, figuring prominently
in schizophrenia, the disturbances of borderline and narcissistic
conditions (Rinsley, 1982, 1985), and sexual perversions. Yet it is
also true that such representational differentiation is relative and
that even in health the pre-object dimension of our experiential
world is operative. In this sense self- and object representations are
never completely differentiated or separated from one another.

The complex interrelationships of self- and object representations have long been a subject of study by psychoanalysts and

---

An earlier version of this chapter was published under the title "The Shadow of the
Object: Notes on Self- and Object-Representations" (Kumin, 1986). The title is similar
to that of Christopher Bollas's book *The Shadow of the Object*, and a few words of
introduction are perhaps necessary. The original version of this chapter was written
in 1982, prior to my introduction to Bollas's work, and was first published in
Psychoanalysis and Contemporary Thought in 1986. Both my paper and Bollas's book
take their titles from a crucial passage of Freud's that is apposite to our central theme:
the ways in which the prestages of object relationships are internalized as aspects of
self-experience. I refer to Bollas's work in this revised chapter and elsewhere in this
book.

developmental psychologists. After the achievement of self- and object constancy such representations are generally thought of as being differentiated or pure entities, that is, stable mental images of one's self *or* of one's objects. However, the ongoing pre-object dimension of experience assures that they are in another sense hybrids or composites. An understanding of the pre-object foundation of experience teaches that the vicissitudes of both self- and object representations are normally so intertwined as to make their firm differentiation occasionally problematic.

In this chapter I will develop the idea that a certain degree of fluidity of self- and object representations is not necessarily of pathological significance but is in fact a ubiquitous developmental process that derives from pre-object relatedness and is essential to healthy object relationships. I will trace the basis for such a view in the psychoanalytic literature, describe certain aspects of the subject from the point of view of developmental psychology, and explore some of the clinical implications of this perspective.

SELF- AND OBJECT REPRESENTATIONS AS COMPOSITES

Recent developmental research seems to indicate that the infant's perceptions alternate between calm states in which the idiosyncratic expressions of emergent self-experience has relatively free play (Sander, 1983) and more emotionally labile states in which the representations of self and objects are merged. The infant becomes increasingly capable of differentiating itself from its mother and other loved objects until, at approximately the end of the third year of life, it has developed a relatively stable internal sense of its own identity in its mental, emotional, and physical aspects, as well as a stable sense of the separate and continuing existence of others (Mahler, Pine, and Bergman, 1975).

This permanent sense of others has been called object constancy, and the sense of one's cohesive self-experience has been called self-constancy. The terms are misleading, however, since they refer neither to the actual self or object nor to actual constancy. For example, object constancy refers to the stability and permanence not of the external object but of the internal mental and emotional representation of the object. By the same token, self-constancy refers not to the ongoing existence of the physical self, which requires bodily intactness, but to the emotionally stable organization of self-representations and self-experience (Kumin, 1978a, 1985). Hypothetically, one could experience self-constancy despite gross physical impairment or even disfigurement and, conversely, suffer severe deficits in self-constancy in the presence of normal bodily health. By the same token, object constancy can be achieved despite the absence or death of the original objects. More precisely, then, the terms are not meant to describe constancy of the self and object per se but constancy of the self- and object *representations*.

Such "constancy" is not actually constant, though. Mahler and her colleagues (1975) stated that the achievement of self- and object-representational constancy is relative and that these representations continue to be refined and differentiated throughout life. Even in the most mature individuals the capacity for fluid shifts and transformations is still retained. In love, for example, the representations of self and object oscillate between states of differentiation and states of fusion (Kernberg, 1977). Empathy, to cite another example, requires an ability to temporarily inhabit in fantasy the feeling states of another individual. Further, as I will describe later, such ubiquitous mental processes as identification, projection, and projective identification also dynamically transform the constancy of self- and object representations from moment to moment.

In several essays Freud (1905, 1914b, 1917a, 1921, 1923) addressed the duality of object relations and their economic vicissitudes. He indicated more than once his view that the ego and its objects are complex entities whose energy and composition are interrelated and in some ways interchangeable. In "Three Essays on the Theory of Sexuality," for example, Freud (1905) wrote that the finding of an object is actually a refinding of it, an allusion to the lost primary object. The period of Freud's greatest concern with these issues occurred immediately prior to the introduction of the structural theory and shortly thereafter, when he was forming his view that the ego is a kind of living membrane posed between the internal and external worlds. In "Mourning and Melancholia" Freud (1917) described the alterations not only of cathexes but also of the representational components of object relations. He wrote that in the melancholic an object cathexis is replaced by an identification: "Thus the shadow of the object fell upon the ego, and the latter could henceforth be judged as though it were . . . an object, the forsaken object. In this way *an object-loss was transformed into an ego loss*" (p. 249; emphasis added). In "The Ego and the Id" Freud (1923) wrote, "The character of the ego is a precipitate of abandoned object cathexes and . . . it contains a history of those object choices" (p. 29).

Freud seems to be saying that a reciprocal relationship exists between the ego and its objects in terms of their internalized economic and representational vicissitudes. Economically, the cathexis of the object representation could be partially derived from the narcissistic cathexis of the ego, and the cathexis of the ego could be partially derived from what were originally object cathexes. Representationally, the object representation is constituted in part along the lines of the self-representation, and the self-representation (an ego function) is constituted in part along the lines of the object representation. This developmental paradox obviously intrigued Freud and culminated in his dual usage of the German term "*das Ich*" to signify the ego as both the experiencing subject and also as the whole person, or object of awareness (Laplanche and Pontalis, 1973).

Chasseguet-Smirgel (1985) added a developmental dimension to this formula when she asserted that the primary object is only later experienced as an object. The "finding of an object" Freud refers to in "Three Essays" can be thought of both as a dimension of archaic object relatedness (a refinding of a lost part of the pre-object mother) as well as a dimension of narcissistic experience (a refinding of a lost part of the self). This lack of distinction between self-experience and object relatedness characterizes pre-object states. Self and object are one in the pre-object state not so much because they are symbiotically merged as because they are intermodally linked. Khan (1979a) introduced the concept of the "collated internal object," which he asserted is involved in the development of sexual perversions. According to Khan, the collated internal object contains elements deriving not only from the actual object but also from the self. But does the pathology of such patients derive from the collated aspects of their object representation or from its relative dissociation from the remainder of their identity and isolation from true object relating and therefore growth? Freud pointed the way to an understanding that even in normal development both the object representation and the self-representation are essentially intermingled. As early as "The Interpretation of Dreams" Freud (1900) wrote that "representation by means of identification" entails, in the dream work, the "construction of a *composite* figure" (p. 321; emphasis added).

In the course of normal development, for example, the self-representation includes not only aspects that derive from the individual baby but also aspects that originally derived from the regulatory system comprising the baby and its caregivers. The mother's expression, the look in her eye, the feel of her holding and cuddling, the tone of her voice, even the infant's perception of that aspect of itself that is the object of its mother's desire (Lacan, 1949) eventually become internalized as the forerunners of autonomous self-caring capacities and are subsequently transformed by the child into aspects of the self-representation. These contributions from the object to the identity and autonomy of the child become narcissistically amalgamated with other aspects of the self-representation, yet there is never an absolute integration.

Pine (1982) lucidly commented on Winnicott's description of the early paradoxical pre-object state in which the infant's mother is experienced as a part of its self and its drives are experienced as part of the external world:

> Thus, ironically, the first (presumed) (pre)self-experiences are brought about by an external agent (the mother); this is the inverse of another irony that Winnicott discusses, that the first *inner* experience, drive pressure (or need), is experienced as an "it" that *happens*, rather than an "I" that *wants*. (p. 147; emphasis in original)

We see the complement of this notion in the observation that the individual's representation of the object is composed not only of his or her relatively objective perceptual images of the object but also of various subjective aspects that have been attributed to the object. Even after the achievement of self- and object boundaries the object is represented both as an externally perceived presence and as an identification merged with the self-representation (Schafer, 1968). Similarly, the self is represented both as a subjective experience and as an internalized object to which we are attached and from which we suffer separation anxiety:

> We are very aware of the infant's dialogue with his real object. . . . But I should like to postulate that we have a parallel process occurring . . . in which the child *constantly and automatically also scans and has a dialogue with his own self to get refueling and affirmation, through the*

perception of cues, that his self is his own familiar self, that it is no stranger to him. (A.-M. Sandler, 1977, p. 199; emphasis in original)

Compton (1985) traced the historical development of the concepts of identification and introjection and concluded that ambiguity in these concepts is related, in part, to ambiguity in the terms *ego* and *object.* I would add to this conclusion the assertion that these concepts are confused partially because the developmental lines of self- and object representations are intertwined and to a certain extent reversible (Kumin, 1978b). While most humans develop a capacity for differentiation between their self- and object representations, these representations are also intermodally linked. Each representation can be thought of as occupying some point along the axis of a self/object continuum (de M'Uzan, 1978).

As I have described elsewhere (Kumin, 1978b), dualistic intellectual systems partly reflect the developmental history of psychic reality. The common tendency to conceptualize in terms of antithetical polarities derives from the persistence of a developmental need for a sense of firmly differentiated existence from the mother. This need is in contrast with the simultaneous narcissistic need for union with the mother, a partially undifferentiated state that, by supporting emergent selfobject functions, paradoxically supports the development of differentiated selfhood. The opposition of these two developmental lines is externalized onto social systems or intellectual constructs and mistaken for an attribute of external reality when in fact it is a feature of internal reality and subsequent ego organization. There are numerous examples of such dualistic systems: In psychology, Freud described the polarities of active and passive, love and hate, and masculine and feminine; in philosophy, one might think of noumenon and phenomenon (Kant) or *en-soi* and *pour-soi* (Sartre); in politics, it might be the dualities of liberal and conservative or East and West; in aesthetics, one might distinguish between form and content. To any such list of ephemeral dualities I would add the concepts of an individuated self and differentiated objects as represented and experienced in one's inner world.

According to Stolorow (1975), since the earliest relationships of necessity maintain the experiential cohesion, stability, and positive hedonic tone of the baby's archaic self-representation, "primitive object relationships and primitive narcissism are two inseparable sides of the same coin" (p. 183). Since the infant and mother at times function in a state of functional inseparability, in the representational world primitive narcissism and pre-object relatedness are also inseparable. These characteristics of the representational world are normally retained into adulthood and are, in fact, crucial for the maintenance of mental and emotional health. De M'Uzan (1978) stated unequivocally:

> No doubt, the mother never stops being a narcissistic object and likewise the ego is never altogether separated from the non-ego. On this basis one may ask whether highly cathected objects can attain the real other-ness of an independent subject. . . . Nor is the ego, partially lost in the image of the objects it invests, able to attain a full identity. Strictly speaking, there is no fixed boundary between the domains of ego and non-ego, but merely a transitional space. (p. 490)

An apt metaphor is that of atomic structure. Electrons were once thought of as discrete particles revolving around the atom's nucleus much as planets in a solar system revolve around the sun. However, this metaphor turned out to be misleading. The quantum theory enabled us to understand that all particles in motion also have wave properties, and for a particle the size of an electron such wave properties are of considerable importance:

> As a result, the electrons in an atom cannot be pictured as localized in space but rather should be viewed as smeared out over the entire orbit so that they form a cloud of charge. The electron clouds around the nucleus represent regions in which the electrons are most likely to be found. The shapes of these clouds can be very complex, in marked contrast to the simple elliptical orbits of planets. (*New Columbia Encyclopedia*, p. 180)

In addition, electrons, after absorbing a photon of the correct frequency, will "jump" directly to a higher energy state without ever passing in between the two energy levels (Avi Kumin, personal communication, October 1992). There is a similar utility in conceptualizing object relations, both in their endopsychic and in their interpersonal vicissitudes, as having the qualities of both particles and waves, that is, as being both discrete and differentiated psychic images and as being "smeared out" over an intermodally linked self/object field of complex shape. The shape and feel of the field derive from the pre-object matrix of the infant and mother's primary relationship. Thus, representations of self and object, in addition to being thought of as differentiated entities reaching a relatively constant and stable configuration between 15 and 36 months, can also be thought of as complex configurations composed of both self and object elements in dynamic interaction and intermodal exchange with each other throughout life. Affects and sensations "jump" directly between these elements without requiring a transitional space or representational thought. Ogden (1986, 1989a, b) described such interaction and reversibility as a central aspect of mental life: Each aspect of the "dialectical" relationship of one form of object relatedness with another "creates, informs, preserves, and negates the other" (1986, p. 208). The normal gamma-function that yokes self- and object representations is the internalized derivative of the mutually regulatory intermodal exchange between the mother and the pre-object infant.

This self/object field (with the slash mark between *self* and *object* representing an intermodal exchange) occurs as a substructure of each individual self- and object representation, as a continuum between the endopsychic representations of self and object, and in external reality as an interactional field between the individual and other persons. Far from blurring the experience of differentiated selfhood, the shape and feel of this field adds depth, substance, and regulation to the experience of being one's self, just as the third dimension of a stereoscopic image results from the simultaneous perception of a second image from a slightly different perspective. Because of the normal functioning of the self/object field, the experience of differentiated selfhood is stabilizing rather than alienating. The self/object field maintains one's sense of attachment in the face of autonomy; it is the core assurance that one is pre-object related as well as object related. Winnicott eloquently described this developmental milestone when he pointed out that the capacity to be alone derives from early experiences of being alone *in the presence of the mother* (Winnicott, 1958b). After the development of an internal representational world the oscillation and interaction between wholly differentiated (i.e., particle-like) and partially differentiated (i.e., wave-like) modes of relatedness (or, in other words, between object and pre-object relatedness, between alpha-function and gamma-function; or between secondary and primary process) represent a lifelong aspect of all human experience. Human existence occupies some place on a continuum between intrapsychic and

autonomous experience at one pole and intersubjective and reciprocal experience at the other. Each creates, supports, and negates the
other.

THE SELF/OBJECT REPRESENTATIONAL FIELD

If one rolls a ball to a child, the child will roll it back. This entails no
reversal between self- and object representations and maintains
what I would call "natural perspective" between subject and object.
Natural perspective occurs when the subject experiences himself or
herself primarily as a self-representation and experiences the object
primarily as an object representation; it is a hallmark of object
relating. I emphasize the word *primarily*, since I have already established my view that once the representational world is established,
"pure" self- and object representations (e.g., an object representation
not perceived in any way subjectively and a self-representation that
contains no influence of the interaction of significant others with the
self) do not in fact exist.[1]

While much attention has been focused on the *reaction* of
infants to external mirroring (Kohut, 1971, 1977; Lacan, 1949;
Winnicott, 1960b), less attention has been drawn to the mirroring
action of children. Infants between 8 and 10 months are adept at
gestural imitation. Gestural imitation differs from the cross-modal
imitation abilities of neonates because it is a *conscious and voli-
tional* mimicry. If the adult opens his mouth, the baby will do the
same; if the adult smiles, the child smiles back. Yet when the adult
waves good-bye to the infant, we notice a curious phenomenon: The
infant waves also but frequently does not wave to the adult. Instead,

---

[1]Winnicott (1963a) once emphasized that "in health there is a core to the personality
that . . . never communicates with the world of perceived objects" (p. 187). This
"incommunicado element" serves as the substrate of the core sense of self. While, at
first glance, the statement seems to contradict my contention that all representations
are alloys, I find in retrospect that my views are in part an outgrowth of this paper
of Winnicott's. Winnicott emphasized that the isolated core does not communicate
with *perceived* objects, thus implying that this central experience of the self originates
in developmental periods antedating the individual's capacity to perceive the object
as an object, that is, as external to the self. Such a capacity to perceive objects requires
the formation of an internal representational world. In short, the core of the self is
rooted in the normal intermodal aspects of pre-object functioning, aspects that are
prerepresentational. The core of the self is incommunicado in the sense that it cannot
be fully represented in purely mental terms.

infants wave with their palm facing themselves, just as the palm of the adult faces them. While such imitation probably indicates the child's lack of capacity to understand the meaning of the gesture, an additional observation is salient. In this instance the child's gesture is not like a mirror image of the adult's but is identical to the adult's gesture from the child's point of view. In terms, then, of the representational configuration of the child's gesture, one is led to the conclusion that that aspect of the child's "representation in action" (Piaget and Inhelder, 1969) has *reversed perspective* by way of an intermodal exchange and become equivalent to the adult's gesture of waving.[2]

Children who are beaten will sometimes hit themselves or otherwise act self-destructively. Such identification with the aggressor (A. Freud, 1936) is illustrative of a clinical situation in which the object representation reverses perspective with the self-representation. The child abuses himself or herself as if one aspect of his or her self-image had itself become the battering object. Projection and identification are the prototypes of mental processes that display the characteristics of reversed perspective. In identification the self-representation "is modified on the basis of another (usually an object) representation as a model" (Sandler and Rosenblatt, 1962, p. 137).[3] In projection the reverse occurs: The object representation is modified on the basis of some aspect of the self-representation. In the subjective world, identification makes the self like the object and projection makes the object like the self. Both entail a reversal between self and object components of the individual's phenomenal world. Further, these reversals are not always static but may often be in dynamic interaction with each other (Green, 1978) based on intermodal exchange. Projective identification, for example, involves a two-way reversal of perspective: The "metabolization" by an external object or internal object representation of projected aspects of the self-representation and the later reinternalization of these now "detoxified" aspects as part of self-experience (Bion, 1959; Grotstein, 1985; Malin and Grotstein, 1966; Ogden, 1979, 1982).

---

[2] Bion's (1963) use of the term "reversible perspective" describes a kind of resistance employed by certain adult patients through which the meaning of the analyst's interpretive efforts is nullified. As such, his concept refers to a phenomenon different from what is discussed here.

[3] The representation used as a model for identification can also be based on a fantasy.

Rather than being thought of as different mental processes, projection and identification can thus be thought of as reversible aspects of the *same* mental process by which the pre-object foundations of experience are transformed into mentally representable object relationships. Projection and identification achieve an equilibrium between the *representational* poles of self and object. Similarly, projective identification achieves an equilibrium between the *interactional* poles of one's self and one's others, inside and outside. Projection and identification operate within an intrapsychic, representational identity field whereas projective identification operates in an interpersonal, interactional identity field.[4]

Strictly speaking, introjection is not a process in which representational reversal occurs. In keeping with Sandler and Rosenblatt (1962), I use the concept of introjection in "a restricted sense to refer only to the processes of transfer of authority and status from objects in the 'external' world to the superego in the 'internal' world, as described by Freud in the *Outline*" (p. 132). Because of introjection, a child reacts in the absence of the parents as though they were still present. Sandler and Rosenblatt give as an example of introjection "the child who obeys a parental injunction (in the absence of the parents) not to stay up late, even though the parents habitually do so themselves. If he identified with the parents, he would stay up late" (p. 138).

Since the representational world develops out of an innately structured pre-object matrix in which infant and mother communicate via reciprocal and regulatory intermodal equivalence of action, gesture, thought, and affect, the boundaries between self and object are at times experientially blurred and the boundary between introjection and identification is not always clear-cut. In the example given by Sandler and Rosenblatt, it could be said that either decision, to stay up late or go to bed early, is based on an identification, although with different parts of the parents' personalities. To use the metaphor of the mind set forward by the structural theory, if the child goes to bed late he has identified with his image of his parents' egos (or, if he imagines it is exciting to stay up late, with his image of their ids), whereas if he goes to bed early he has identified with his image of his parents' superegos. What then is an

---

[4]Similarly, empathic attunement and other forms of intermodal exchange also operate in an interpersonal and interactional identity field.

introject? A more interactional way of conceptualizing an introject might be as an individual's identification with his perception of an object's representation (or *mis*representation) of him. Such identifications with parental projective identifications have an unconsciously "not me" experiential quality that differentiates an introjection from the "me" experience of a true identification.

In any event, both self- and object images contain elements of each other—components that are of reversed and nonreversed development. Further, the whole realm of transitional phenomena may be viewed as an equilibrium between ego and object, natural and reversed perspective; a simultaneous intermodal exchange between self and object; a null point in the intertwined developmental processes of introjection, identification, and projection. Put another way, representational reversal is an *effect*; intermodal exchange is its *cause*.

While reversal is primarily a vicissitude of the representational world, it is also a mode of object relating as well as the prototype for certain ego defenses. The personalization of the infant is achieved in part through its primary maternal identification as well as its later identifications with others. Similarly, the infant's personalization of its object world and the development of a sense of intersubjectivity is partially achieved through the projection of attributes of the self-image. Children become able to put themselves in another's shoes, to understand and be considerate of another's feelings, to do unto others as they would have others do unto them.

Once the child has developed a subjective internal world, each drive derivative, whether conscious or unconscious, is associated with a self- or object representation (Fairbairn, 1952; Kernberg, 1966; Sandler and Sandler, 1978; Stolorow and Atwood, 1979). Since all drives and affects contribute representational components to the subjective images of self and object, all defenses against the drives and their derivatives alter the representations of self and object.

The consequences of such changes ultimately become manifest in the psychoanalytic situation. Certain defenses, such as repression, displacement, reaction formation, undoing, and rationalization, alter the mental representation of drives and drive derivatives while tending to retain natural self/object perspective. For example, if the patient at a given moment resents the analyst and defends against the associated drives by praising him or her, we call this way of dealing with psychic conflict a reaction formation. In phenomenological terms the patient has defensively altered a hateful self-image into a loving self-image and has simultaneously altered a hated object representation into a loved one. This transformation primarily affects the drive component of the representation of the object relation, turning hatred into love. In this alteration there is no self/object reversal; natural perspective is maintained. If in addition the conflict concerning the analyst is a repetition of a childhood conflict with a parent, we would describe this defense as a displacement of a representation from a past object relationship onto a current one. Natural perspective is still maintained.

Conversely, other defenses, such as projection, identification, and projective identification, primarily alter the representations of self and object by reversing their perspective. Take, for example, a person having conflicts over his or her own sexual desires. Motivated by a need to defend against such an awareness, the individual might disapprovingly attribute those same unbridled desires to some minority group. The projection does not change the representation of the drive—which remains sexual—but reverses the location of such drives in the representational world. Rather than the sexual impulses being perceived as aspects of the self-representation, they are experienced as an aspect of some object representation.

> A patient who fit in many ways the description of a "false self" related a particularly vivid and instructive experience: He had been camping one weekend with his wife. She decided to photograph him while he posed near a river bank. As she was adjusting her camera, the patient noticed a water moccasin near his foot. To his later amazement he found himself unable to jump away. As he reconstructed his experience, he felt incapable of moving until his wife also saw the snake. But she was busy focusing the camera and adjusting its aperture, and he felt bound by her wish that he remain still. Eventually, she did notice the snake with a start, and then the patient instantly jumped away.

Transference is generally thought to entail a defensive displacement of the representation of a past object or object relationship onto the image of a contemporary object or object relationship. This customary way of thinking about transference emphasizes the central role of displacement, which preserves natural representational perspective. However, the concept of transference may be usefully expanded to include a place for identification and projection, which reverse representational perspective.

Lipton (1977) described a specific type of transference resistance utilizing identification as the chief defense. He gave as an example of this type of transference a patient of his who while exiting his office at the end of the hour turned to him at the door and said in a detached way, "Well, that was a wasted hour." In analyzing her statement during the subsequent session, Lipton concluded that in fact the patient had found the hour to be quite a good one but had imagined that he had, with some detachment, considered it to have been a wasted hour. Lipton noted that the same sort of identification may also be interpolated among the associations of a session rather than added as an afterthought. He cited as examples instances of the patient interjecting comments such as "This all seems like nonsense," "I don't know why I'm wasting my time on this," or "It seems as if I keep going over the same things." The patient defensively reverses self/object perspective by modifying his or her self-representation along the lines of his or her fantasy of the critical analyst.

Another representational transformation occurs when the "object" displaced or projected in the transference is a self-representation (Meissner, 1981). This occurs (1) during an idealizing narcissistic transference, as described by Kohut (1971, 1977), where a grandiose self-representation is displaced onto the analyst; (2) in certain transference psychoses occurring in the treatment of borderline patients; and (3) also in a more benign and transitory way in all analyses. Such transference-based projections occur whenever patients do not explain sufficiently what they are talking about because they assume the analyst understands what they mean or when patients assume the analyst is motivated by conflicts similar to their own, or is of the same religion or shares the same political beliefs or taste in music.

In fact, one frequently finds both a self and an object component occurring simultaneously in the psychoanalytic situation, each of which requires interpretation for full resolution to occur. Langs (1976, 1977, 1978a, b) was a pioneer in drawing attention to the bipersonal (Baranger and Baranger, 1966) elements of the psychoanalytic situation, in its interactional as well as its intrapsychic elements. He described a "me/not me interface" as being intrinsic to all psychoanalytic communication and advised that all statements of the patient be understood as a potential commentary about the analyst as well as the patient.

Transference can thus be thought of as not only (1) the displacement of an object representation onto the analyst, but also (2) the identification of a self-representation with the analyst, (3) the projection of the self-representation onto the analyst, and (4) an intermodal exchange and reversibility between patient and analyst that is not fully representable in symbolic mental terms. Only the first-mentioned (i.e., classical) usage of the concept of transference entails a solely natural perspective; the last three involve a reversal in the experience of self and object. The first three aspects of transference are qualities of object relatedness while the last aspect is a quality of pre-object relatedness. Thus, one of the results of psychoanalytic interpretation is not merely the returning to consciousness of disavowed aspects of the patient's self- and object representations but the *creation of representability* of aspects of self-experience that previously could not be "thought" about or experienced directly. This leads to an increasingly differentiated and natural perspective to the patient's representational world.

The following chapter discusses in greater depth the traumatic absence of representation and its psychoanalytic creation (not *re*-creation).

CHAPTER SEVEN

Creation
of Representability

P RE-OBJECT RELATEDNESS is a forerunner of the capacity for
mental representation. It stands to reason, then, that any
trauma, developmental arrest, or inborn disturbance that impairs
pre-object relatedness disrupts the infant's capacity to form mental
representations. Thus, one of the results of psychoanalytic interpretation is not merely the returning to consciousness of aspects of the
patient's repressed unconscious but the *creation of representability*
of aspects of self-experience that previously could not be "thought"
about or experienced directly because of infantile disturbance. The
past catastrophe is simultaneously unrepressed and yet unthinkable.

Such a purpose of psychoanalytic treatment is of considerable
importance in the psychoanalytic treatment of those individuals
whose disturbed early relatedness has resulted in functional impairment of the capacity to form mental representations.

A woman in the first few months of analysis began a session
feeling depersonalized, unreal, and out of touch with her own
feelings. After I pointed her disturbance of affect out to her and
invited her to think about its source, we traced its onset to a
brief experience prior to the beginning of the session. She had

---

Portions of this chapter were presented to the Seattle Psychoanalytic Society on
March 6, 1989, and to the Northwest Alliance for Psychoanalytic Study, Seattle, on
June 16, 1990.

walked by the open door of my office on her way to the rest room and saw me working at my desk with my back turned to the door, unaware of her presence. She realized that she could not fully be aware of herself because I had not been aware of her; she could not fully feel she existed subjectively until she was confident she existed for me. Further, until that moment she had no conscious awareness that she felt I had let her down in any way. We traced this vulnerability not only to her mother's advanced Alzheimer's disease but also to much earlier disturbances in her parents' emotional recognition of her moods and needs.

I do not think that the patient's feelings were repressed in the usual sense: that is, symbolically represented but actively kept out of her awareness. As far as I could tell, her feelings were not yet attached to thoughts or symbols, even unconsciously. Her feelings, as manifested in the session, were concrete, psychosomatic, prerepresentational. Only when I put my patient's needs into words for her, when I said that she could not be aware of her own feelings as long as she felt that I was unaware of her, did genuine emotion creep into her voice and was she able to think about and experience her wishes and feelings.

During my work with another patient, a severely depressed woman, I was again impressed by the clinical utility of bearing in mind that psychoanalytic work not only lifts repression but also creates representation. Soon after the start of her psychotherapy she became mostly silent in her sessions, a state that lasted the better part of two years. None of my ways of understanding silence seemed to apply to this woman. Interrupting the silences to ask her what thoughts or feelings were going through her mind would invariably prompt her to answer, "Nothing," after which she lapsed again into silence. Accepting her silences as a sign that she was not feeling safe enough to speak and allowing them to continue only made matters worse and deepened her sense of futility and hopelessness. My interpretations proved ineffective and usually incorrect.

The patient's silences did not seem to be merely symptomatic of the profound depth of her depression. At first I considered them to be pervasive resistance to therapeutic involvement. I assumed that when she said she was thinking of nothing, she meant this only metaphorically. That is, either she feared that I would think she was not thinking about anything I would be interested in or she feared my response to what she was thinking would be seductive or retaliatory or she herself was thinking about something sexual or aggressive or she wanted to provoke some mood in me with her silence or she just did not want to tell me what she was thinking about for some purpose I could not yet fathom. However, when I attempted to interpret her behavior along these lines, my interpretations were met with a heightened sense of despair and failure, and more silence. She would glance around my room with what appeared to be mild interest, but she rarely looked at me and then only briefly, in passing. I thought that it was as if, from her point of view, there were a hole in the room where I was sitting. However, I considered this an idle fantasy of mine, so the significance of this observation was not available to me for quite a while. In the meantime, the patient's depression seemed to be worsening ominously.

Very gradually I came to understand that, my patient, unlike those whose words convey symbolic or metaphorical meanings, meant what she said literally. She was in fact thinking of nothing, and the nothing she was thinking of was not symbolic but concrete. There were never any people in her dreams, no living creatures of any sort, no feelings or speech, only vectors of force and direction. Nor was there an observing self. In other words, the nothing she was thinking of did not stand for something else or hide anything else; it was a thing-in-itself. In contrast, Lewin (1948b) described a neurotic patient who claimed to be thinking of nothing as a way of symbolizing unconscious fantasies about female genitalia and castration anxiety. My patient's nothing did not mean anything else; its effect was to extinguish meaning.

Two years later I found some support for this view when I came across Sidney Klein's (1980) paper formulating the presence of what he called autistic barriers in nonpsychotic patients. Klein drew upon Frances Tustin's work with autistic children as well as Wilfred Bion's description of certain states of severe neurosis that conceal a psychotic part of the personality. Klein wrote:

> These autistic phenomena are characterized by an almost impenetrable encapsulation of part of the personality, mute and implacable resistance to change, and a lack of real emotional contact either with themselves or the analyst. Progress of the analysis reveals an under-

lying intense fear of pain, and of death, disintegration or breakdown. (p. 400)

I was intrigued by the similarity in Klein's description of an impenetrable encapsulation of a part of the personality and my description (Kumin, 1978a) of schizoid states as representing the hypertrophy of what Freud called the "peripheral rind" of the ego as a protective "outer shell" to a fragmented and poorly structuralized ego core. In a series of studies that relate to these ideas, Tustin (1986) described the use by autistic children of "autistic objects" and "autistic shapes" in order to delineate their own body surfaces by tactile sensations. She stated that their activities "are mostly asymbolic. They do not play, dream, fantasize or imagine to any appreciable extent" (p. 124). Unlike schizophrenic or symbiotic children, who feel filled with terrifying primitive internal objects, autistic children are in a largely objectless state. The external nonhuman "autistic objects" used by such children,

> are not objects in the true sense; they are hard, object-like sensations engendered by grasping an object tightly. They are pseudo-objects in that, like the soft autistic shapes which are engendered by holding an object loosely, they have no existence apart from the child's own manipulations. They do not exist in space and they have no spatial relationships with other objects. They have no shared meanings. They are peculiar and personal to the child alone who, by touching them, brings them into being for his own idiosyncratic purposes. They are inseparable from the sensations they engender. (p. 146)

According to Tustin, such affectively sealed-off concrete states can also be found in hard-to-reach adult patients who would not otherwise be considered psychotic. Ogden's (1989a, b) description of "autistic–contiguous" aspects of experience has enlarged our understanding of the effects of these earliest experiences in the treatment of adult patients.

Kinston and Cohen (1986; Cohen and Kinston, 1983), in a series of highly original and clinically relevant papers, maintain that mental representation in the form of a wish is the result of having one's needs met. Failure of need mediation in infancy leads to persistent absence of representable wishes, a condition Freud alluded to in his concept of primal repression. This failure of need mediation is traumatic and leads to a "persistent wound," a "gap" in emotional understanding, a "hole" in the fabric of experience. They assert that "hole repair is what psychoanalytic therapy is about" (Kinston and Cohen, 1986, p. 337). Because such occurrences are not represented, they are not repressed.

> It is precisely because repressed unconscious experiences are *represented* . . . that they can appear in dreams, slips of the tongue, symptoms and so on and can be brought into consciousness by interpretation. By contrast, the (non-represented) trauma that constitutes primal repression cannot be simply observed or experienced by the analysand or brought directly to his attention by interpretive comments. (Kinston and Cohen, 1986, p. 338; emphasis in original)

However, at the beginning of my silent patient's treatment I did not understand these issues well. It was only after many painful months of therapeutic impasse that I finally conveyed to her my tentative new understanding that her silence might not be a type of avoidance but a direct communication of her oppressive inner emptiness. She immediately appeared relieved, and her depression lifted somewhat. A session or two afterward she reported a dream which I considered confirmatory.

> *In the dream she was being inexorably pursued by an invisible creature that was coming to kill her. She frantically tried to hide from the "nothing monster" while simultaneously protecting and shielding a young child.*

The patient then began talking occasionally in sessions. She still required prompting from me (her words were sporadic and isolated), but usually when she did speak, she spoke with what I felt at the time was intense depth of feeling. Over the course of the next few months I became increasingly aware of something I had not noticed at first. It was a peculiar way she had of speaking. She would describe some interaction with another person that would have aroused an intense reaction in anyone, yet she blandly and factually presented the information shorn of adjectives, devoid of emotion, and lacking even first-person pronouns. I had been wrong when I previously thought the patient was speaking with intense emotions. She was *suggesting* the presence of painful affects to me while not yet feeling them herself. The depth of feeling I perceived had in fact been evacuated from her; her tone of voice and facial expression remained detached.

In one session the patient claimed that she was not avoiding her feelings, that she just did not have any. I said to her that her absence of feeling was a way of erasing herself, that she considered nonexistence to be the ultimate protection from emotional pain. In the next session the patient looked and felt better. For the first time, I noticed that she was smiling in the waiting room, and she reported her first dream in months:

> *The scene of the dream was depicted on a computer screen that was gradually being turned to white as the cathode rays scanned back and forth across the screen from top to bottom.*[1] *The entire dream was becoming blank, as if the glass picture tube displaying the dream was being spray-painted white from within and was becoming an opaque barrier. The patient said it seemed that the dream itself was dissolving into a fine white mist on the screen. She sensed that the obliteration of the dream could be total and permanent. Somehow, she took action by frantically typing in some commands at the computer's keyboard and was eventually able to stop what was happening. She woke up terrified.*

Now, the patient and I had previously come to a sense of conviction that when she was six months old, she had lost a significant element in her mother's care and attention. This occurred because her mother's mother suffered a breakdown and moved into the patient's home, where she received constant attention from her daughter (who was a nurse) while she received a lengthy course of outpatient shock therapy. The patient's mother became severely depressed herself while she assumed the responsibility of caring for her mother, and in a significant way she was lost to her baby, my patient.

But beyond this early loss, and perhaps emblematic of it, there was something else about the patient's mother that disturbed the patient throughout her life: The patient was convinced that her mother did not hear her when she talked, that she was somehow

---

[1]Rosenfeld (1987, p. 176) described a dream with a similar manifest content that was reported by a patient of his.

listening past her. It was as though her mother could only hear what she wanted to hear. The only way the patient could relate to her mother was through compliance, or so she felt. Anything else the patient said did not register, it did not exist, for her mother. The patient and I explored the ramifications of this feeling in the transference, including the possibility that I might be like her mother, given the length of time it had taken me to understand her and to hear her. On the day before the dream, however, she *had* felt understood by me, and it was this understanding that created a capacity for her to represent what had previously been erased, that enabled her to have this particular dream and remember it.

TWO DIMENSIONS: THE DREAM SCREEN

I took notice of the cathode ray tube that bore the representations of the dream, an image that in one sense might have derived from her sense of detachment from her feelings. But the plane of the computer screen that was being erased by beams of cathode rays reminded me of Lewin's (1946) twin concepts of the dream screen and the blank dream. Isakower (1938), writing about regressive hypnagogic phenomena associated with falling asleep, believed that the sensation of large masses approaching the dreamer represents breasts. Lewin hypothesized that the same process occurs in reverse as the dreamer awakens, with the breasts receding into the distance as the sleeper reestablishes ego boundaries. This idea was based in part on Federn's (1952) assertion that the waking ego reconstitutes itself along the same lines that prevailed in its development, a process Federn called "orthriogenesis."

According to Lewin, the surface of the breast appears to flatten out and become a plane as it approaches the dreamer and thus becomes the blank background on which all dreams are projected. Lewin (1946) wrote that the dream screen came to his attention when a young female patient reported, "I had my dream all ready for you; but while I was lying here looking at it, it turned over away from me, rolled up, and rolled away from me—over and over like two tumblers" (p. 88).

Lewin's conjecture was that the rolling away of the patient's dream screen was merely the final event in the complete awakening represented by her resistance. In another paper Lewin (1948a) cited the dream of a patient whose dream shattered "like a pane of glass" while receding, leaving the patient with a sense of picking up the pieces. The similarity of that dream to my patient's dream is manifest. On the nature of dreaming Lewin wrote the following:

> The dream screen appears to represent the breast during sleep, but it is ordinarily obscured by the various derivatives of the preconscious and unconscious that locate themselves before it or upon it. These derivatives, according to Freud, are the intruders in sleep. They threaten to wake us up, and it is they in disguise that we see as the visual contents of the dream. On the other hand, the dream screen is sleep itself. . . . The visual contents represent its opponents, the wakers. The blank dream screen is the copy of primary infantile sleep. (1946, p. 90)

Although rare, there are dreams without visual content in which the dream screen appears by itself. According to Lewin (1946), since the blank dream "represents the breast situation in a nearly pure state" (p. 90) and thus provides pure fulfillment of the wish for "union with the mother in visually blank sleep" (p. 91), it typically presages states of elation or hypomania.

While Lewin's hypotheses seemed serviceable to me in understanding certain elements of my patient's partially blank dream experience, other facets of her experience were not confirmed by his hypotheses. Foremost among these was the fact that the dream, far from being a blissful wish fulfillment, signified only a brief respite from crushing depression. The patient had found the "whiting out" of her dream to be a frightening experience and desperately tried to stop the process. While one might speculate that the fearful affect represented a defense against the gratification of a regressive wish, I was inclined to take my patient's report at face value. The wish represented in the dream was the desperate wish to hold on to her representational world, which was in danger of being erased by the deprivation of vitally supporting relatedness. In my patient's case, the dream thoughts and images in the computer were not the awakeners but the preservers of the dream and sleep. It was the threatened loss of the image of herself and the desperate struggle to hold on to that image that was terrifying and that awoke her. The threatened whiting out of the dream screen had been terrifying to my patient, and only the cessation of this process had brought her relief. The representational images, contained within the dream's computer, were reassuring; contrary to Lewin's hypothesis, it was the advancing flattened blankness of the computer screen that was the awakener.

N DIMENSIONS: THE DREAM CONTAINER

Today many would put less emphasis on the infant's instinctual relation to the breast and more on the encompassing role of the infant's relation to the totality of its mother's care. Lewin alluded to these issues when he emphasized that the dream screen is experienced only secondarily as a two-dimensional surface. The dream screen is a flattening of the originally three-dimensional object of the mother's breast as it approaches the infant's mouth, its skin surface filling the infant's visual field. However, in his discussion Lewin focused on the qualities of the dream screen as a plane surface. It is as if Lewin's conception of the infant–mother relationship also became two-dimensional because it allowed a concentration on the breast to obscure its vision of the mother. Three-dimensional models were added with Winnicott's concepts of the transitional space, Bion's dual concepts of the container and the contained, and Spitz's observational studies of infants.

Winnicott (1958a, 1965) wrote that the good-enough mother provides a "holding environment" that supports ego growth. In such a holding environment id experiences strengthen the ego, but in its absence these experiences produce overwhelming states akin to annihilation. When development proceeds within normal limits, a transitional space is created in the internal world, situated somewhere between the infant's experience of the subjective object and its experience of the object perceived objectively. This transitional space can become a dream space.

Bion (1962a, b) described the ordinary mother's capacity for "reverie," through which she is able to be attuned to her infant's signals; "contain" its nonverbal distress, which is communicated via projective identification; and assist the infant in reinternalizing what was previously felt to be overwhelming. Partly due to the mediation of the mother's reverie the infant is able to utilize its own innate capacity to develop alpha-function, which transforms the beta-elements of raw sense impressions and fragmentary ego particles into a more integrated form fit for storage, symbolic thought, and dreams.[2]

Spitz modified Lewin's and Isakower's assumptions, which were based on Freud's theory that the first object in life is the mother's breast. Spitz (1965) noted how throughout the nursing process infants stare fixedly at the faces, not at the breasts, of their mothers until they fall asleep. He suggested that during the first six weeks of life a memory trace of the human face is laid down in the infantile memory as the first signal of the presence of the mother. Subsequently, the infant follows every movement of this signal with its eyes. Accordingly, Spitz suggested that from the infant's point of view the visual aspect of the dream screen does not represent the mother's breast but her visually perceived *face*.

The three-dimensional spatial metaphors of Winnicott and Bion and of Spitz's reconsideration of the sign gestalt aspects of the nursing situation point the way to a further reconsideration of the dream screen from the perspective of the infant's pre-object relations. Even the mother's face acquires no meaning for the infant in the absence of the ego-nurturing and self-structuring support she provides for the infant. The surface of the dream screen—the breast or the mother's face—is given life and enduring meaning by the *totality* of the pre-object relationship between infant and mother, an n-dimensional relationship. It is the infant's anaclitic relationship with its mother and its experience of the totality of the nurturing, need-gratifying, and stimulus-regulating environmental provision by her that provide the backdrop for the images in the dream and the emerging representations of self and object. Thus, if the two-dimensional dream screen, in keeping with Lewin's metaphor, represents the satiating breast (or the sign gestalt of the mother's face during nursing) that provides a return to primary narcissism, then the nth dimensions are added by the mother who responds to the infant's signal, understands the baby's communicated need, and mediates that developmental requirement in a good-enough way. If it is possible to imagine the baby's point of view, the mother's face is a gestalt that acquires meaning because it thinks and feels and responds to the baby's emotions, thoughts, and actions. In addition,

---

[2]In Chapter Four I described this innate capacity—of the infant to utilize its attachment to its mother's emotional understanding in order to develop alpha-function—as a gamma-function that intermodally links infant and mother, beta and alpha.

the mother's breast contains not only milk but the precursors of a whole inner world available for the infant to internalize, and it opens a path that leads toward human relatedness and representational thought. While the relation to the breast initiates a process of ingestion and digestion of milk (which sustains and strengthens the infant's body), the relation to the mother initiates a process of relating to an internalized object that regulates and neutralizes drives (which sustains and strengthens the infant's ego).

Applying these ideas to my patient's dream, I saw that the computer screen she faced opened into an internal world in which the dream was being played out. It was a space in which her self, her mother, and the other important people in her world, including me, were encompassed. This image was being gradually obliterated by a projected stream of electron rays. While this image could be understood in terms of minute particles of projective identification that drained her and threatened to leave her blank and estranged, McClelland's (1993) recent paper on autistic space presents another way to understand the erasing of the computer screen. Describing the way in which the representational world may become "deconstructed," McClelland wrote:

> In thinking of autistic space I am thinking of a mental or psychic state in which many (but not all) of the usual linkages between or within mental representations are relaxed or abolished. In such a psychic environment, the representations become available in a more or less confused and chaotic way. An analogy would be the Brownian motion of very small particles suspended in a free solution or colloid. That is, in autistic space our mental representations become less differentiated than they are normally. (p. 202)

My patient was terrified by her vulnerability to a representational deconstruction perhaps derived from pre-object pathology of relatedness. At an early age she had internalized her mother's deficient awareness of her existence and was therefore blocked in having direct insight into her own thoughts and feelings. Mangham (1981) described the gradual development of insight out of the relationship between infant and mother:

> ["Insight" is a metaphor that is] taken from the experience a child has with his mother. In this experience the child perceives his self, his mother, and the interaction with her as "seeing into" him, and knowing

and understanding what she sees. This perception by the child of the experience with mother is then internalized and experienced by the individual as self-awareness, self-understanding, or seeing into oneself, all of which can be thought of as forms of "insight."

The mother–child process also incorporates the attachment of words to feelings and behavior, and the way this "naming" sometimes results in a feeling of success, a feeling of mastery, and reduction of tension and psychic pain. The mother's "naming" and the analyst's interpreting thus both create meaning—insight—but are also linked by the early affective bond. (pp. 271–272)

Mangham goes on to state conclusively, "In other words, awareness of something within the self is a function of maternal awareness and is a function of the relationship between the mother and her infant" (p. 272).

Furman and Furman (1984) have described temporary loss of the child's ego feeling as secondary to the mother's "intermittent decathexis" of the child. They described how children lose contact with their sense of themselves when they perceive that they have ceased to exist for their mother. Analogously, my patient's chronic decathexis of herself was an identification with her mother's chronic decathexis of her, beginning with her mother's depression during the patient's first year of life. This relationship to an empty object, poorly differentiated as internal and poorly differentiated from herself, led to an oppressive inner feeling of emptiness and alienation. In relation to this empty object the patient was trapped in pre-object modes of experience that predated her capacity for representational thought.

Dowling (1982) reached a similar formulation in describing a patient who also suffered from repetitive blank dreams. After these contentless dreams she would awaken with a sense of dreadful emptiness and terror that was "beyond anxiety." Dowling linked such dreams to disturbances in the primary relationship:

> Viewed developmentally, the defining characteristics of primary process, [that is,] condensation, displacement and symbolization, are different ways of looking at a single mental achievement, representational thought. . . . My patient's imageless dreams, like Isakower's patients' hypnagogic phenomena and Lewin's blank dream and related phenomena, are not true representational thought; they make use of an earlier, prerepresentational organization of mental content. Percepts (organ-

ized sensations), motor recognition (actions which occur with familiar sights or sounds), and affective states are ingredients of this early organization. (p. 161)

Dowling linked this early form of mentation to Piaget's concept of sensorimotor organization and described how the central traumatic experiences related to his patient's overwhelming blank dreams occurred prior to the age of two.

Green (1980) described a massive blank depression developing in the child of a depressed mother. Green's emphasis was on the effect of this experience on the imago of the mother, which is decathected and then used as a model for identification, producing a decathected self-representation. My own understanding is that such massive blank depressions are linked more to pre-object experiences that predate the differentiation of the maternal representation and that, owing to their linkage to trauma that cannot yet be represented, pattern the overwhelming character of the affect along with the blank experience.

Using the theoretical model of attachment theory, Pound (1982) described the severe consequences of maternal depression for the later development of affective psychopathology in children. Main and Weston (1982) described the development of avoidance of the mother as an infant's response to the mother's avoidance of the infant. Indeed, my patient felt her mother's sense of her to be without warmth and authenticity, lifeless, two-dimensional, unfeeling, static, without animation, computer-like. This experience then was felt to be a part of herself, what Green described as a "cold core." My patient had identified with the missing mirror image of herself she saw in her mother. The patient's inability to get through to her mother (and now to others, including me) created a hole in her experience. This early deprivation that was just beginning to be represented was the "nothing monster" that relentlessly hunted her, the glitch that threatened to erase her representational world. She felt in constant danger of being erased as a person and, by identification, of erasing herself. She then became able in her dream to avoid becoming blank because of her relation, in the transference, to me as a primary object able to contain an accurate perception of her.

As Kinston and Cohen (1986) pointed out, however, the establishment of primary relatedness, characterized by "intense mutual attachment and deep empathic communication" (p. 343), creates hope and risk. The risk jeopardizes the continuation of the treatment and is often represented by what appears to be serious deterioration, suicidality, or life-threatening illness. While there is debate on this point in the literature, Kinston and Cohen (1986) emphatically stated that the risk, being real, often requires the analyst to act in a far more direct and less exclusively interpretive manner than usual: "The direct care . . . involves actively valuing and accepting the analysand, recognizing and reflecting his experiences, and being intensely attentive and concerned even occasionally to the point of action on behalf of the patient—in other words finally allowing primary relatedness to manifest" (p. 346).

Potentially lethal risk requiring direct care manifested itself one day when I sensed with great concern, at the end of a session, that my patient was about to make a suicide attempt immediately after leaving my office. I anxiously called a family member in another city, the only person she had mentioned whom I knew how to reach. The family member immediately called a friend in town who rushed to the patient's apartment to check on her. When the friend arrived, the patient was just opening a bottle to swallow what would have been a lethal number of pills. She had said nothing to me about her intentions in the preceding session, not even in derivative form (as far as I could consciously recall). I am still not certain how I knew. Was it the expression on her face? My own uncharacteristically sharp feelings of hopelessness, pessimism, and failure as her therapist during that session? The finality in her voice as she said good-bye? And if it was the latter, how did I know what was for her the tone of finality?

By the end of this patient's treatment, three years after the computer dream, she had internalized the capacity to understand her own meanings as an ability to appreciate herself. She was able to love and to work. She returned to school, completed the studies she had all but abandoned, applied for postgraduate training, entered and enjoyed a stable relationship with a man, and, not least of all, was able to talk with me spontaneously during her sessions.

In one of her last sessions she told me about a frustrating situation at work that was reminiscent of her dream three years earlier. The situation at work, which seemed to be an unconscious metaphor for her views about the source of her depression and the result of her therapy, was this: The patient had been stymied that morning because the host computer on her network had not recognized her account number. As a result, she was not able to load and run her software. She had, in effect, been shut out of the networked communications. After describing the situation to me she fell silent for a few moments, a pause that at the beginning of her treatment would have signaled the start of a shattering blank depressive crash. This time, however, she brightened, smiled, and said, "But it was okay. I figured out that I could get access to my data by borrowing someone else's account."

CHAPTER EIGHT

The Container of Sleep

THE VIGOR OF a psychoanalytic concept as a way of usefully organizing clinical experience derives in part from its evocativeness as a metaphor. One such metaphor, that of the container in which intrapsychic contents are imaginatively elaborated, has had a compelling effect on contemporary psychoanalysts. The concept of a psychic container was first systematically developed by Wilfred Bion; since then it has been employed widely by a diverse range of authors, including Shengold (1985), Loewald (1988), Chasseguet-Smirgel (1988), Modell (1988), and Anzieu (1989), who have developed the idea in ways that, if not always in reference to Bion or true to his original intent, considerably broaden the appeal and explanatory power of his concept.

Despite criticism of the reification inherent in the idea of a mental envelope, its appeal as a metaphor is considerable. The recent attention to the psychic container has both derived from and led to thoughts about the psychoanalytic situation and its holding and containing functions, the nature of the therapeutic alliance as a background for the progressively unfolding transference, and the role of the analyst in the development of more adaptive ego functions in the patient. Anzieu (1989) clearly summarized the implications of this emerging understanding: "Psychoanalysis presents itself . . . as a theory of unconscious and pre-conscious psychical contents. . . . But a content cannot exist without some relation to a container" (p.

Portions of this chapter were presented to the Seattle Psychoanalytic Society on March 6, 1989, and to the Northwest Alliance for Psychoanalytic Study, Seattle, on June 16, 1990.

11). Calling the shift in attention from psychic contents to the psychic container an "epistemological about-face," Anzieu wrote, "The forms of pathology with which the psychoanalyst is increasingly faced in his practice today derive in large part from disturbances of the container–content relation."[1] According to Anzieu, the analysis of such disturbances must offer the patient "an inner disposition and way of communicating which [holds out the] possibility of a containing function and allow[s] him to interiorize such a function sufficiently" (p. 11).

Anzieu's question of how the patient interiorizes a replacement for a previously deficient containing function during psychoanalytic treatment inevitably leads back to a study of pre-object mental states, and especially to an interest in the relationship of the infant to its mother and to her body. Chasseguet-Smirgel (1985, 1988) claimed that patients may have a variety of transference reactions to the psychoanalytic situation itself, each based on the patient's relation to the interior of the mother's body as container. For example, if the patient's unconscious wish is to destroy the contents of the mother's body, then there is also hatred and intolerance of the contents of both the analyst's mind and the patient's own mind (in identification with the analyst/mother) as well as an intolerance of the frame of the psychoanalytic situation.

It is this aspect of pre-object relatedness that I address in this study of the internalization of a containing function in the development of dreams.

THE ERASABLE DREAM

In "Dream as an Object," J.-B. Pontalis (1974) set forth the hypothesis that "every dream refers to the maternal body in so far as it is an object in the analysis" (p. D5). Pontalis suggested that the dreamer shares with the child clutching his security blanket a

---

[1]There are certainly similarities between the container–contained object relations metaphor deriving from the oral psychosexual phase and the container metaphor deriving from the anal psychosexual phase (Shengold, 1985). Because of this, the question sometimes arises in reconstructing clinical pathology as to whether these metaphors derive from the first or the second year of life. In fact, there is often a dual derivation from both phases since there is a developmental line of the container–content relation originating in pre-object states.

common element: Neither can bear to be separated from that link to the mother that symbolizes, and at the same time makes real, her absence.

It is my suggestion that it is not by making the mother absent that the dream connects the dreamer to her; the dream links the dreamer to the mother *because* she is sensed as being absent. She is lost through sleep and found through the dream. And further, it seems to me that it is not so much the mother's body per se that the infant seeks for discharge but the *stimulus-regulating functions that are embodied* in the concerned holding and containing provided by the good-enough mother. In this regard the infant's increasing internalization of the homeostasis-maintaining functioning of the infant–mother pair provides what Grotstein (1985) has described as a "background object of primary identification."

The originally containing object is the affectively attuned mother who provides her infant with a sense of her as an interior holding not only milk but reverie (Bion, 1962b).[2] This interior, whose location may not initially be differentiated by the infant, may also be experienced as providing an envelope in which to collect nascent experiences of the self. The experience of a container provides cohesion for ego nuclei to coalesce.

Freud (1923) was explicit that the ego "is that part of the id which has been modified by the direct influence of the external world" (p. 25). Writing about how the ego is ultimately derived from bodily sensations, chiefly those springing from the surface of the body, he asserted that the ego is "first and foremost a bodily ego; it is not merely a surface entity, but is itself the projection of a surface" (p. 26). However, one becomes aware of the surface of one's skin— and thus aware of an ego boundary, in Federn's (1952) sense—when and where it touches something or is touched. The ego in this sense has a double surface, an interface between the surfaces of self and object functioning as a semipermeable membrane. Freud (1925) was the first to note the double-layered surface of the ego in "A Note upon the 'Mystic Writing-Pad.'" He considered the outer layer to be a protective shield and the inner layer to be like a "writing surface" for the storage of memories. In this sense, the infant becomes

---

[2]While I personally would place the development of this sense of an inner space quite early, my concern in this discussion is not the precise timing of the development of this sense but merely the acknowledgment that such a sense does develop in time.

preconscious when it comes into contact with an object. The object contact that generates thought and feeling can be emotional as well as physical, and it has a valence. The touch can be warm or cold, secure or insecure. The object that is contacted may be both animate or inanimate, and it may be a part of the infant's own body. Hoffer (1949) called attention to the considerable implications for ego development of the "double touch" of one part of the infant's body with another. This might occur, for example, during finger sucking, when the interior of the infant's mouth contacts its own hand, or when the infant plays with its own fingers. Charles Mangham (personal communication, March 1989) pointed out how this double experience of touching and being touched by one's self serves to organize early experiences of the self and aids in the beginning differentiation of self and object, active and passive.

If the ego is ultimately a projection of the skin, then ego functions develop in part through the projection of the double skin surface where the infant touches and is held by the mother. Thus, there is, corresponding to Hoffer's "double touch," a double projection, outward and inward, simultaneously calling into existence experiences of both self and object on either side of the contact surface between the infant and its object. Since, as I discussed in Chapter Six, projection and identification are aspects of the same process, there must also be a double identification at the contact surface making objects human and the self recognizable as one's self. Thus, as described in an important paper by Bick (1968), the emotional functioning of the mother, as well as her empathic mental capacity, creates the experience of a binding mental skin. The enveloping mental sac provided by the mother creates a surface for projection and identification when it comes into contact with her infant and enables the infant to experience a mental skin of its own. Anzieu (1989) has gone so far as to refer to the ego as a "skin ego":

> By Skin Ego, I mean a mental image of which the Ego of the child makes use during the early phases of its development to represent itself as an Ego containing psychical contents, on the basis of its experience of the surface of the body. . . .
>
> From this epidermal and proprioceptive origin, the Ego inherits the dual possibility of establishing barriers (which become mechanisms of psychical defense) and filtering exchanges (with the Id, the

Super-Ego and the outside world). . . . As a further consequence, then, the Skin Ego underlies the very possibility of thought. (pp. 40–41)

It is as if the interior of this physical and mental skin surface created by the holding and containing mother is an n-dimensional holographic screen on which representational thought and dreams are projected and identified. This is a process similar to intermodal perception and representation across sensory boundaries. The quality of the infant's sensorimotor contact with its mother brings into existence preconscious physical and mental representations. The infant gradually internalizes the mother's concern, indeed, all of the physical and emotional components of the mother's care. The mother's mind is "taken in," as surely as her milk. The internalization of the mother's body (physical touch: milk and holding) and mind (emotional touch: affect attunement and reverie) is necessary for the relief of hunger and other overwhelming physical discomforts, as well as for the relief of overwhelming affect states.

FROM THE SIDE OF THE INFANT: THE CONTACT BOUNDARY

The infant internalizes its mother's capacity for being cognitively and empathically matched to it as a functional ability to regulate and neutralize its own drives. The infant's internalization in depth of its relationship with its mother enables it to create an internal representational world that feels warm, alive, real, and deep. This representational world then becomes utilized in the service of dream work. Qualities of the interaction with the mother are integrated as components of a sense of self and as integrators of the synthetic activity of the ego. But how might this occur?

When Freud (1923) wrote that the ego was a precipitate of abandoned object cathexes, he was ambiguous as to how we are to think of the object. Is it an objectively perceived person or the subjective mental representation of that person, permeated by the individual's wishes, fantasies, feelings, defenses, and motivations? If we think of the object as a person, then Freud would seem to mean that the forces that once attached the infant to the mother and other loved ones eventually serve as strengtheners of the ego. If, however, we mean the object in its mental and emotional sense, then something more subtle is implied. The implication then is that the capacity to find and bring to life an enduring object representation (i.e., object constancy) leads to an equivalent finding and animation of the self as a stable and secure experiential structure able to generate effective and modulated action. I would make clear here my view that while the infant is biologically predetermined to develop ego functions and affects, it is the emotional component of the infant–mother pair that lends to that internal world its signature tone and quality.

Overwhelming stimulation produces both intense affect and muscular discharge states in the neonate. The mother helps to shield the baby from excessive levels of stimulation. She serves as a protective shield for the infant in the sense that she assists the infant to regulate its involvement with the inner and outer world. The excessive stimulation may be of efferent or afferent origin: internal, as when the infant is hungry or exhausted, or external, as when the infant is cold or bombarded by loud noises. The stimulation may also be from emotional sources of both internal or external origin.

While the infant is awake, tension reduction is mediated by muscular discharge. The overstimulated infant screams, turns red, kicks, and thrashes frantically; it violently tries to rid itself of the overwhelming sensation. One interpersonal effect of such behavior is to signal to the mother the need for some soothing and adaptive behavior toward the infant. A second effect, an intrapsychic one, is that the violent physical and emotional discharge forces the infant to generate what I would call a contact boundary. The thrashing infant forces its body to contact either the human or nonhuman surfaces that surround it or initiates emotional contact with an object by signaling its need for an interactional response from the caretaker. When the physical or emotional sensation of contact is experienced, it is as if a mental surface, the forerunner of an ego boundary, is experienced.

The contact boundary serves as a node around which nascent ego functions precipitate, such as a sense of personal existence, the possession of interior mental space, and the sense of cohesion of self-experience. Federn (1952) was the first to study the boundary functions of the ego. Later, Bick (1968) not only described how the early adaptive responses of the mother enable the infant to achieve the physical sensation of being bounded by a physical and mental skin but also linked pathology of this skin experience to psychosomatic illness. More recently, Tustin (1980, 1984, 1986, 1990) and Ogden (1989a, b) have explored the primitive containing function of the ego's bounded surface. It is plausible to assume that this surface feels alive, that it in fact has many feelings, and that it is therefore linked to affects. In some sensorimotor way it might be experienced as waxing and waning, as continuous or instantaneous, as located here or there, and as fully surrounding and containing the infant or as porous. The contact boundary maintains a bounded surface that is felt to contain self-experience. As described earlier, the contact boundary, having two sides, is sandwiched by the forerunners of self- and object representations, as well as by the possibility of an internal and external world. To the extent that overstimulation from whatever cause is unbearable for the baby, it also is unendurable. When the infant's effort to establish a contact boundary fails, the wait for relief must seem endless and thus may also seem to collapse the beginnings of the infant's awareness of time.

While it is considered controversial to attribute sophisticated motivational patterns to the infant at such an early stage of development, it is not necessary to postulate that the infant perceives the separateness of the object or intends to achieve contact with it. One need only consider that the effect of the baby's response to overstimulation achieves this end, the establishment of a contact boundary, and that the boundary effectively demarcates self, object, affect, time, intentionality, and other nascent ego functions for as long as it exists.

DREAM WORK AND PROJECTIVE IDENTIFICATION

Freud (1900) believed that dreams are the guardian of sleep because they provide hallucinatory wish fulfillment and thus reduce drive tension. The origin of dreaming would then seem to coincide with the first existence of mental representations, whenever that occurs and in whatever primitive form they exist. Because dreaming seems to occur during states of paralysis of the large skeletal muscle groups, it requires the mental representation of muscular discharge and containing contact for tension relief in order to preserve sleep. According to Tahka (1987), "The sensations associated with tension reduction . . . being recalled as hallucinations are likely to be the organism's first efforts to master tension by psychological means" (p. 236).

Holt (1967) questioned whether the occurrence of REM sleep and other psychological indicators of dreaming, like penile erection, in neonates indicates anything resembling the adult type of visual dream. He postulated that "the physiological sleep- and dream-cycle is . . . [an] innate given . . . into which content can be put when and only when the capacity to represent absent objects develops" (p. 377). Holt's phrase "into which content can be put," while certainly not originally intended as a metaphor for the processes described here, is nevertheless apposite. I would postulate that just when a primitive mental self that can dream is being formed, a dream object is created to replace the absent mother. The dream object guards sleep. The contact boundary between this forming object and forming self might have a hallucinated double skin surface. Since the boundary between self and object is not fully differentiated in the dreaming state, the contact boundary might be experienced as something like a "double touch," corresponding to Hoffer's conception, described earlier, in which the infant plays with its own fingers and simultaneously experiences itself as touching and touched, self and object. The infant's experience of the interior of this object (which, owing to incomplete representational differentiation, the infant would also imagine to be its own interior) would provide a sense of a soothing container and a screen surface for the infant's projections. Freud (1917) emphasized the role of projection in dream formation when he wrote the following:

> The final outcome is that the sleeper has dreamt and is able to go on sleeping; the internal demand which was striving to occupy him has been replaced by an external experience, whose demand has been disposed of. *A dream is*, therefore, among other things, *a projection*: an externalization of an internal process. (p. 223; emphasis in original)

The "internal demand" is for the lost relation to the tension-relieving and stimulation-regulating mother. Like flickering shadows on the walls of Plato's cave, projective hallucinations would correspond to Holt's "content" representing the relation to the regulatory object. Such an experience of being contained is required in order to preserve sleep in the absence of the mother, the original guardian of sleep.

Mental representations of the mother thus help to structuralize the emerging self-representation of the infant and moderate its raw emotions. This process also occurs in reverse. The infant's projections enable the mother to seem more reassuringly familiar and understandable and facilitate the internalization of a structuralized representation of her. The two processes are interwoven in that a self that is beginning to be differentiated and differentiating, neutralized and neutralizing, is better able to perceive and experience the object and to dream about her.

From the perspective of the double projection at the contact surface that is the dream screen, it could be said that dreams guard sleep because the dream not only is felt to be contained by the self but also represents an object that is felt to contain aspects of the dreamer. In this sense, the dream acts as a modulator and channeler for internal and external stimuli during sleep. Sandler (1960a, 1987b) discussed this function of the dream work:

> In sleep, disturbing stimuli from any source may be dealt with by the dream work, and in this sense we can regard the dream not only as the guardian of sleep but also as a perceptual mechanism that maintains the level of safety feeling within the ego. (1987b, p. 5)

The dream screen can be thought of as resulting from the infant's internalization of the mother's reverie against and into which the dream is projected. Just as the mother is the infant's guardian, the dream is sleep's guardian. Accordingly, Bion wrote,

> It used once to be said that a man had a nightmare because he had indigestion and that is why he woke up in a panic. My version is: The sleeping patient is panicked; because he cannot have a nightmare he cannot wake up or go to sleep; he has had mental indigestion ever since. (1962b, p. 8)

By way of example I think of a woman who had been in analysis with me for two years.

The woman had consulted me in part because of a sense of alienation from herself. During her analysis she had been slowly coming to terms with the slow death of her mother and realizing that her estrangement from herself was partly an identification with her half-dead the mother who could no longer recognize her. This reminded her that she had never felt fully recognized by her mother, even as a child. What the future held for her relationship with her mother seemed to replicate her past. As she gradually allowed herself to face these realities, she began to emerge from her cocoon of isolation.

I had canceled a Monday appointment over a holiday weekend with only a week's notice (not my usual practice). The weekend of my absence came and went, and at the Tuesday session the woman said she felt disoriented, confused, detached, and "in a fog." She had felt this way the entire weekend but had no idea why. She said she had not been able to work effectively and had not been able to sleep. Yet she recalled a dream, a rarity for her:

In the dream I had all kinds of really gross bugs inside of me, like maggots. There was some kind of container that was clear, you could see into it, and it had chemicals inside of it. By using it, it would draw the bugs out of me and they would die. Someone gave me the container and instructed me how to use it. I was supposed to hold it up to my chest and it would draw them out of my chest into the container. I had to use it several nights in a row.

Among the many meanings the patient and I eventually discovered in her dream was the idea that I had been providing a means for her to rid herself of the awful feelings and conflictual wishes inside of her. While these specific contents were analyzed subsequently, it was the nonspecific containing and mediating *function* that first required understanding and restoration in the analysis. The container was transparent—a narcissistic object; the patient had only a transitory awareness of the object *qua* object. I was represented only by my pre-object function, as an object delimited only as an outline, a boundary that provided cohesion for projected and identified aspects of her self. (I should add that this symbol of the container was her own; I had never used the word before in the analysis.) This function she felt I provided, this receptiveness, this neutralization of all the gross things that were "bugging" her, had been disturbed by the unpredictability of my absence. When the patient was able to acknowledge and consciously experience the emotional effect of my loss on her, her functional capacity to work and sleep returned and her mood improved.

Thus, fluctuations in the quality of dream affect and dream symbolism during analysis may in part reflect not only the internal state of the patient's drives and conflicts but also the patient's perception and experience of the quality, tone, and developmental level of the analytic "holding environment." We know that the ego's symbolic function has a developmental line, epitomized by the progression during latency age from nightmares about amorphous monsters to animals to humanoid figures. In analysis the symbolic capacity may also regress or progress as a reflection of fluctuations in the state of the internal containing object. This ego function depends on factors intrinsic to the self as well as on the nature of the transference, the actual analyzing function of the analyst, and the security of the patient's attachment to the analyst in the analytic situation. The patient's perception of disturbance in the analyst's capacity to contain the patient's anxieties through empathic attunement and accurate interpretation undermines his or her own containing ego functions (Kumin, 1989). The perceived functioning of this internalized object that supports self-regulation may also be affected by the nature and quality of the patient's projections. The felt loss of the containing object threatens an actual loss of or regression in the self-regulating ego functions it supports. This increases the likelihood of projective attempts to reestablish the containing experience.

The patient's dreams may shift from more affectively neutral dreams about whole objects in conflict to more affectively raw dreams invaded increasingly by nonhuman part-object figures such as reptiles, insects (like the aforementioned patient's maggots), or more primitive creatures (like the invisible monster of the patient in the previous chapter). If the internal containing functions fail, dreaming itself may be troubled, sleep is disturbed, and acting out may ensue as projection via enactment becomes a more pressured way of seeking external contact boundaries and containing receptacles for the overwhelming affect state. Kelman (1975) claimed that in the treatment situation actualization of the manifest content of dreams is most likely to occur during points of greatest stress in the transference and countertransference, suggesting that the analyst's capacity to tolerate the patient's affect states decisively influences the patient's containing functions.

In a journal article L. Grinberg (1987) discusses the containing function of dreams from a similar perspective. He proposes (Grinberg, 1987) a clinical classification of dreams during the analytic process, with dreams that elaborate and work through at one extreme and dreams that evacuate at the other, and also views evacuative dreams as involving a search for an external object who will serve as a container. Grinberg (1987) writes, "Animals, machines, or apparatus from outer space, nonhuman elements, partial objects, usually appear in the manifest content of these [evacuative] dreams. The dreams often coincide with gross alterations of the setting, severe acting out behavior, or serious somatizations" (p. 160).

I would also add that in the most extreme form—the complete dehiscence of the internal container—this process results in regression to prerepresentational mentation manifested by terrifying blank dreams, states of bewildering emptiness, imageless panic, and other manifestations of pre-object developmental trauma.

SELF-DESTRUCTION AND A DEATH DREAM

The reestablishing of an internal containing object is frequently noted in a progressive shift in the quality of dream symbolism or in the renewed capacity to dream when dreaming had previously not been possible.[3] It is no coincidence to regularly find a marked increase in remembered dreams before and especially after the analyst's vacations in patients in the middle phase of analysis, and Grinberg and Grinberg (1960) have discussed the importance of "Monday dreams" after the weekend separation from the analyst. Monday dreams in this sense represent a reconstitution of the analyst's containing functions in his or her absence, as was described in the discussion of the container dream of my patient. This point suggests to me a dream that seemed to signal an early turning point in the analysis of a panicky and suicidal woman:

> The woman had sought help in part because of her fear that she would be unable to stop herself from hurting her young child while she was in a state of rage. She had herself suffered real

---

[3] I am, of course, not referring to the physiological function of dreaming during REM sleep that occurs every night but to the capacity to remember analyzable dreams.

physical abuse during her adolescence. In a Monday session, which had been preceded by a rare panicky weekend phone call, she described a series of recent actual abandonments and abuses by people she depended on. Unstated was the abandonment represented by the weekend break from analysis. The patient described losing her temper with her daughter and slapping her hard enough to knock her over. She immediately felt overwhelmed with guilt and wanted desperately to cut her own wrists, as she had done once before, prior to the analysis. During the session she was extremely anxious, on the verge of tears, and distraught.

I said something about her intense feelings related to being the passive victim of abuse by others, including me. This intolerably overwhelming feeling had been a central concern of the analysis; not a great deal was new in what I was saying to her. I added that she needed to protect herself by converting her feelings into a form of active abuse, directed either against herself or her child, and that she felt it was preferable to be the abuser than the abused.

She thought about this without much conviction. After a while she angrily remembered the early days of her treatment, when I saw her in psychotherapy because I could not arrange to begin her analysis immediately. She recalled a comment of mine made during that initial period and asked me if I remembered saying that I thought that analysis would eventually be of help but that, in the meantime, she would have to hold the situation together. "Well," she asked, "*how am I supposed to do that?*"

There ensued a long and uncharacteristic silence, during which I felt an intense and almost overwhelming pressure to say something. At the same time, I felt at a complete loss for anything useful to say. Fortunately, I was able somehow to resist the temptation to blurt out something meaningless just to rid myself of the awful feeling. I was able to hold my own internal situation together long enough to realize that the shoe was now on the other foot, so to speak, and that I must be having an inkling of how the patient felt. My feeling of internal pressure immediately disappeared. Accordingly, I said, "It sounds as though you're saying that when you feel this way, it's impossible for you to contain the feelings and you must act upon them."

At her next session the patient was much calmer and immediately said that she had a dream the night before. (This was her first dream in over two months.) In the dream she was told by a female physician that she was suffering from leukemia, the "childhood type," and that she might only live a week. The doctor gave her some pills to take q.i.d. (we were meeting four times a week). The doctor seemed seemed unsure if the pills would work but told the patient to give them a try. The patient, however, was relieved by the diagnosis. As she told me, "Leukemia was what I wanted."

The patient spoke spontaneously about wanting to die, but the difference was that she was talking *about* her feelings rather than being overwhelmed by them. I reminded her that she had felt hopeless the day before about containing the devastating feelings she was having and said that today she seemed calmer. She nodded and said, "I *am* calmer." I added that she was able to dream about her feelings rather than having to act on them by hurting herself or her daughter. She was able to have a dream *about* wanting to die rather than actually being on the verge of cutting her wrists.

In retrospect, these two sessions seemed to me to mark the point after which the patient's dangerousness to her self and her daughter began to abate rapidly. The dream indicated that she had been able to begin to internalize a neutralizing function modeled on my ability to both contain her overwhelming affects and transform them into interpretations she found useful. Some time later she said to me, with a new sense of insight and resignation, "I've been depending on someone who isn't dependable." I took this statement to refer not only to me or to those who had recently let her down—and not only to her father and mother, who had abused her during her childhood or had allowed her to be abused—but also to a part of herself who had identified with the abusing or neglectful parent. Now she was beginning to feel that she could depend on herself and that her daughter could depend on her as well.

Her realization also signified that the original environmental failure had now returned to the environment. Before, it was being kept always alive internally as a pre-object part of herself that was incapable of shielding her from traumatically overwhelming stimuli. The deficient internalized care of her body had led her to abuse her own body as well as her child's. Now, despite occasional regressions to overwhelming feelings, the analysis was proceeding satisfactorily in terms of personal wishes, hatreds, and desires, all of which now felt tolerable and safe because they were beginning to be mediated by her own self.

At the penultimate analytic session the patient spoke for most of the hour about beginning to learn a male friend's hobby—rock climbing. She described a method of "roping up," which meant that even if she lost her grip she was roped to the climber above her and would not fall. On one particular day she had felt frightened because her friend was teaching her how to climb a practice rock without being roped. I said that climbing without a rope was like ending the analysis. She thought about this awhile and then added an interpretation of her own: "I think that analysis was like working *with* ropes for the first time in my life. You can go a lot higher if you work with ropes."

PART THREE

Pathology of
Pre-Object Relatedness

CHAPTER NINE

Two Disturbances
of Pre-Object Relatedness

EVEN AFTER THE DEVELOPMENT of object constancy one's representational world normally retains aspects of its pre-object relatedness. Despite the ability to clearly differentiate one's self from others, the mental images of both self and object nevertheless remain composite unities throughout the life cycle rather than "pure," or monadic, entities. Self- and object representations, despite their differentiation from each other, are complex configurations which are "smeared out" over a self/object continuum of complex shape. Projection and identification achieve an equilibrium between the representational poles of self- and object representations, and intermodal exchanges achieve a regulatory balance in the interactions of two individuals. As such, projection, identification, and projective identification are reversible aspects of the same intermodal process by which affect states are transmitted and object relations are represented. It follows, then, that the optimal development of these processes in any individual rely not only on his or her innate genetic competence but also on the regulatory competence of the reciprocal infant–mother attachment.

In this chapter I review seminal studies of early attachment by Mary Ainsworth, Renata Gaddini, John Leopold Weil, and Stanley Greenspan and draw parallels to Robert Langs's observations of forms of adult communicative health and pathology as manifested in what he calls the "bipersonal field" of the psychoanalytic situation. Each of these researchers focuses on a particular age group: Weil on infants, Gaddini on three-month-olds, Ainsworth on one-year-olds, and Langs on adults. The infant studies lack longitudinal follow-up into adulthood, and Langs's theory lacks a developmental perspective. Nevertheless, I hope that a review and juxtaposition of this research may help to fill in these gaps by demonstrating intriguing and significant similarities in the conclusions drawn by the researchers despite different research populations, different data-gathering strategies, and different theoretical orientations. In particular, the weight of these studies leads to the conclusion that there are two central organizing pathologies of affect regulation that are observable in infancy, in childhood, and in the psychoanalytic situation.

THE "STRANGE SITUATION"

In the 1960s Mary Ainsworth, operating from the point of view of attachment theory, studied the patterning of infant attachment from an experimental design she called the Strange Situation. In a series of experiments (Ainsworth, 1985; Ainsworth and Wittig, 1969; Ainsworth et al., 1978a, b) Ainsworth and her coworkers observed attachment behaviors that have far-reaching importance for understanding both the development of fundamental security or insecurity in object relationships and the related health and pathology of an infant's affect-regulating capacities. Long-term follow-up has demonstrated that the effects of early disturbance in the regulatory interactions of the infant–mother dyad are lasting and influence the patterning of character structure and psychosomatic functioning. Since the first descriptions of the Strange Situation were published, the framework of Ainsworth's studies has been employed fruitfully by other infant researchers (Main and Stadtman, 1981; Main and Weston, 1981; Main et al., 1985; Sroufe, 1985; Waters and Deane, 1985; Waters, Vaughan, and Egeland, 1980), although the implications of her research findings have not as yet been fully integrated with psychoanalytic theory and practice.

The Strange Situation has a complex structure that is summarized in the list below. In Ainsworth's pioneering studies the infants were between 50 and 52 weeks old (i.e., after the development of stranger anxiety), and they were tested with their mother, who in each case was the infant's primary attachment figure. Each mother received instructions in advance, generally during a home visit. She was informed of the purposes of the procedure, was told what to expect, and was briefed about her role in the experiment. During the experiment the baby and mother are led into an unfamiliar room containing a chair for the mother, a chair for the stranger (who, in these experiments, was a woman), and toys for the infant.

1. The observer introduces the mother and the baby to the room in which the experiment takes place, then leaves. This takes half a minute.
2. The mother does not participate while the baby is free to explore; if necessary, the mother stimulates the baby's play after two minutes.
3. The stranger enters the room. The stranger is silent for the first minute and converses with the mother during the second minute. In the third minute the stranger approaches the baby. When the third minute ends, the mother leaves unobtrusively.
4. This first separation episode lasts three minutes, or less if the baby is unduly distressed. During it, the stranger adapts her behavior to that of the baby.
5. The stranger leaves and the mother returns. This first reunion episode also lasts three minutes. During it, the mother greets and/or comforts the baby and tries to settle the baby again in play. This episode is prolonged if more time is required for the baby to become reinvolved in play. The mother then leaves, saying "bye-bye."
6. The second separation episode lasts three minutes, or less if the baby is unduly distressed.
7. The stranger enters and gears her behavior to that of the baby. The separation from the mother continues for another three minutes, or less if the baby is unduly distressed.
8. The mother enters for the second reunion episode. She greets the baby, then picks the baby up. Meanwhile, the stranger leaves unobtrusively.

The baby is presented with a succession of situations in which it is alternately left with the mother only, with the mother and the stranger, and with the stranger only. The baby's reactions to the presence of the stranger, the loss of the mother, and the reunion with the mother are observed. Ainsworth and her coworkers observed three general types of attachment behavior: one type in which the infants seemed to be developing optimally and two pathological types.

Secure Attachment

The group of babies who are securely attached (Group B in the report by Ainsworth et al., 1978a, b) are those whose histories are consistent with healthy development. These babies seem confident that their mothers will be emotionally and physically available to assist them if they encounter a frightening situation. The babies show little or no distress during the separation episodes, eagerly seek proximity and contact with their mothers when they return, and endeavor to interact with them. These are intrepid and confident babies, eager to explore the world. Bowlby (1989) claimed that this pattern is promoted by "the ready availability of the parent, in the early years especially the mother, sensitive to the child's signals and lovingly responsive when he seeks protection, comfort, or assistance" (pp. 249–250).

Ambivalent Attachment

The second group of babies, this one demonstrating an ambivalent attachment (Ainsworth's Group C), conspicuously resist contact and interaction at certain times, while at other times they anxiously seek out proximity to and contact with their mothers. Main and Weston (1982) wrote that these infants are "often distressed even before the first separation, fearful of the stranger, and extremely distressed on separation. In general, they seem immature and their response to the Strange Situation seems regressive and exaggerated" (p. 39). The infants seem to display decidedly mixed feelings about their mothers, and their behavior is characterized by anger, separation anxiety, clinging, and hesitancy in exploring their surroundings. Bowlby (1989) attributed the behavior of these babies to parents whose response to their babies is unpredictable, that is, responsive and helpful at some times but not at others. He further believed that this type of insecure attachment is also created by experiences of separation and by threats of abandonment used as punishment.

Avoidant Attachment

The third group (Ainsworth's Group A) is characterized by strong avoidance of the mother in the reunion episodes.[1] The babies either ignore or otherwise avoid their mothers by averting their gazes, moving past their mothers, or turning away. Importantly, unlike that of the ambivalent group, this behavior is *not* angry during the Strange Situation, in that these babies neither cling to their mother nor push her away when picked up. When picked up, they often indicate their desire to be put down in an emotionless way. Main and Weston (1982) noted that these babies, while not expressing anger in the Strange Situation, *do* often express anger toward their mother at other, stress-free, times. The anger appears "out of context" in the form of attacks on the mother that seem unprovoked and inexplicable: "The baby is creeping across the floor, smiling. Suddenly he veers toward his mother, strikes her legs, and creeps away" (p. 42).

The mothers report that these babies often inexplicably hit and bang toys, have tantrums, actively disobey commands from either parent, and act "troublesome." During the Strange Situation they tend to treat the stranger with less avoidance than the mother and show little distress when the stranger is present. These babies preferentially gravitate to the toys and other elements of the non-human surround; have difficulties in social responsiveness to friendly gestures from other adult caregivers outside of the Strange Situation; and are impassive and pseudo-self-sufficient, as if they have no expectation that adults will be helpful or responsive to their needs. There is no evidence that avoidance is correlated with disturbance in cognitive or other types of functioning, and at birth there appear to be no significant abnormalities of avoidant babies as compared to secure babies (Waters et al., 1980). Main and Weston's (1982) observations of infants and mothers indicate that this pattern

---

[1]Some degree of avoidance is a common finding. For example, Main and Weston (1982) observed at least mild gaze aversion in 80 percent of all babies upon reunion with their mother. However, the babies in Group A manifested intense and characteristic avoidance reactions, clearly distinguishing them from other infants.

of avoidance of the attachment figure upon reunion is highly associated with the mother's behavior. They found that the infant's
avoidance is highly correlated with the three qualities of their
mother's behavior toward them: the mother's aversion to physical
contact, her angry and threatening behavior, and her restriction of
emotional expressiveness.

Aversion to Physical Contact

Main (1977) reviewed Ainsworth's original records for the first year
of life and rated the mother's aversion to physical contact with their
infants during the first three months of life. The mother's aversion
to physical contact during this high point of pre-object development
was highly correlated with the infant's avoidance of the mother at
the end of the first year. Importantly, an infant's early "cuddliness"
seems to have no relation to the later emergence of avoidance (Main,
1977; Waters et al., 1980). Main noted not only the mother's expressed attitudes toward physical contact (such as "Don't touch me!"
or "I have always hated physical contact") but also her behavior
during videotaped play sessions (Main and Stadtman, 1981; Main,
Tomasini, and Tolan, 1979).

The Mother's Angry and Threatening Behavior

The mothers of the avoidant babies in the Main and Weston (1982)
were significantly angrier than other mothers, even in the presence
of video cameras. Mothers of mother-avoidant infants mocked their
infants or spoke sarcastically to or about them; some stared them
down. One expressed irritation when the infant spilled imaginary
tea. Ratings showed a strong association between avoidance and
maternal anger in this sample. In addition, in this study significantly more of the mothers of avoidant babies handled their babies
roughly than did mothers of secure infants.

Restriction of the Mother's Affect Expression

Main and Weston (1982) found that the emotional restriction applied to emotions of either pleasurable or unpleasurable valence.
Mothers of babies with avoidant attachment neither registered
pleasure nor changed expression when their babies attacked them

physically. The researchers described the mothers' response as appearing more like "detachment" or "stiffness" than "bland unresponsiveness." Such mothers do not effectively receive their baby's signals for comfort or protection. According to Bowlby (1989), these babies expect to be rebuffed; he attributed the later development of clear psychopathology to this group, including personality disorders manifesting compulsive pseudo-self-sufficiency and persistent delinquency.

PRECURSOR OBJECTS

Since studies relating to the Strange Situation describe insecure attachment in one-year-olds as the outcome of disturbance in mother–infant relatedness, one is naturally led to studies of such relatedness in even earlier developmental phases.

Renata Gaddini studied psychosomatic symptoms such as rumination and colic in three-month-old infants. She drew on the work of the Rochester school, especially Greene (1958) and Engel (1962), a group of theorists who related psychosomatic disturbances to the quality of early object relationships. However, her chief influence for this study was Winnicott's concept of precursor objects. In her chapter in a book on transitional objects and phenomena, Gaddini (1978) begins with a review of Winnicott's concept of the transitional object, an example of which is the baby's "security blanket." The transitional object is that one item the infant habitually utilizes for self-soothing and security, especially at bedtime and other instances of separation from the mother. Winnicott emphasized that the transitional object is not a symbol (although it is a prestage in the formation of the symbolic function). It does not stand *for* the mother, since its difference from the mother is as important to the baby as its similarity. The transitional object is in between subjective and objective reality; it simultaneously assists the baby in maintaining a sense of attachment while enabling early movements in the direction of separation and individuation.

The transitional object is discovered by the infant in the environment during the second half of the first year of life. Gaddini observes that the transitional object usually develops out of the wrapping blanket in which mothers swaddle their babies when nursing. She notes that babies born in autumn and winter months most often have woolen transitional objects while babies born in spring or summer months most often have linen or nylon objects. However, prior to the discovery of the transitional object, the infant utilizes what Winnicott (1967a) termed "precursor objects." Precursor objects, as described by Gaddini, are "those objects, that, while they have the capacity to console the child, have not been discovered or invented by the child. They are provided by the mother, or are parts of the child's or the mother's body" (p. 115).

The concept of a precursor object should perhaps be distinguished here from the concept of pre-object functioning. Pre-object functioning refers to primary forms of relatedness that predate the formation of the autonomous cognitive structures necessary for the ability to maintain the stable mental images of differentiated self and object. Pre-object relatedness is therefore a generic term; it characterizes any of a variety of "preautonomous schema" (Sandler, 1960b) for the later development of "whole" object relationships. It is as if all pre-object relations contribute to a plan or blueprint for the later capacity for the subjective awareness of being an individual with an ongoing sense of a cohesive self, in relationship with other people who are mentally differentiated and emotionally enduring. In this sense, then, the use of a precursor object described by Winnicott and Gaddini is one type of pre-object functioning, although by no means the only type.

Gaddini asserts that the early development of psychosomatic symptoms can be considered as a form of pathology related to failure or arrest in the development of the transitional object, particularly in the prestage of precursor object (which she abbreviates as "P.O.") formation. Gaddini differentiates two basic forms of pathology, represented in Table 9.1. The most severe form of pathology, created by profound difficulties in the infant–mother relationship, results in severe dysregulation of early physical functioning and is later manifested by interactional withdrawal, self-rocking, and incapacity for creative play. The baby attempts to adapt to the failure by premature ego development and self-mothering. This leads to profound withdrawal from relatedness to the actual mother and severe disturbance in development of the self. According to Gaddini,

> If the child is let down all the time, at a later stage self-rocking or other rhythmical body movement will appear. The rocking child

TABLE 9.1. Pathogenic, Borderline, and Facilitating Environments: Their Effects at Two Stages of Development

Environment	Mother	Infant	Early somatic response	Later response
Pathogenic	Not available Not predictable Feeding not a reciprocating event Doesn't get to know her infant Separated from infant in nursery	Let down Apathetic Nonprotected transitions between sleep and waking, hunger and satiation Doesn't get to know mother	Vomiting Screaming crying Constant sleep	No transitional object Nonrelating child Self-rocking Annihilated Psychotic No capacity for creative playing No abstract symbolization
Borderline	Spoils with untimely frustrations Resents dependence	Let down at times Resents nonavailability Untimely experience of frustration	Regurgitation Three-month colic Sleeping difficulties Dermatosis	Language difficulties Masters meanings of symbols principally on somatic level Psychosomatic symbolization
Facilitating	Knows her infant Adapts to infant's needs Frustrates when necessary	Knows mother Transitions clear between sleeping and waking, hunger and satiation	Extending world Development of transitional object or phenomena	Intermediate area between psychic reality and external reality Symbolic functioning Cultural experiences Creativity

Note. Reprinted with permission from Gaddini (1978, p. 126). Copyright 1978 by Jason Aronson, Inc.

imitates his mother: but in so doing he feels annihilated, *becomes* a mother who rocks babies, losing himself in the process. Self-rocking is a sign of deprivation, the result of an inadequate maternal response to his earlier screaming and crying. Screaming, in fact, *is* a cry for the mother, and implies there is still hope. (p. 125; emphasis in original)

A more subtle form of pathology, which Gaddini terms "border-line," is created by "asynchronous" infant–mother interaction and results in colic and difficulty sleeping:

> Colic is the earliest example of an organized psychosomatic disorder of infancy. It can occur by the third month if the infant has not developed a P.O. (the into-the-mouth type particularly), or if the P.O. the child has been provided (pacifier) or has found for himself (thumb, fingers, tongue) is not sufficient to absorb the anxiety stemming from the unbalanced interaction between him and his mother. (p. 119)

According to Gaddini, the borderline environment is not characterized by unending failure of the mother–infant relationship but is nevertheless plagued by intermittent, unpredictable failures in "good-enough" experiences. She continues, "The basic difficulty, however, lies in the mother–child relationship: third-month colic is a somatic response to rage, the infant's 'answer' to the experience of his mother's asynchronous unavailability" (p. 124; emphasis added).

Gaddini's descriptions support the conclusion that disturbances in early affect regulation and psychosomatic functioning are closely related to pre-object pathology, that is, pathology in infant–mother relatedness prior to the infant's development of the capacity for mentally differentiated object relationships. The pathology of the infant–mother relationship is internalized by the infant as a disturbance in the psychosomatic functioning of the self (Taylor, 1987, 1992, 1993). The severity and duration of this internalization is left open by Gaddini's study, however. While the implication is clear that Gaddini considers the two forms of pathology she noted to be prototypes of enduring disturbance in character formation and psychosomatic integrity, the study itself focuses on a narrow time span. Some degree of corroboration is provided by Ainsworth's research on older babies, who show strikingly similar psychopathology. For example, one is led to wonder to what extent Ainsworth's Group C infants, who anxiously seek out proximity as well as avoid it, have internalized the unpredictable lack of adaptation of Gaddini's "borderline" environment. Similarly, Ainsworth's Group A babies, who avoid the attachment figure because of their expectation of maternal unresponsiveness and rejection, show striking similarities to the babies in Gaddini's "pathological" environment.

The findings of Renata Gaddini's and Mary Ainsworth's studies, then, lead to similar conclusions. Competence in the way a mother interacts with her infant is highly correlated with competence in psychosomatic and emotional functioning of the baby, whether the baby is studied at three months of age (Gaddini) or at approximately one year (Ainsworth). Future, disturbance in the way a mother and her baby interact seems to become translated by the baby into enduring forms of psychopathology that affect mental, emotional, and psychosomatic functioning. The pathology appears in both studies to be of two distinct types: one characterized by intermittent outbursts of poorly modulated rage and the other characterized by profound withdrawal from relatedness to others and a precocious but essentially counterfeit self-sufficiency.

"HYPER" AND "HYPO" STATES OF BEHAVIOR

Weil (1992) researched the effects of early deprivation of empathic maternal care while at the Judge Baker Guidance Center in Boston and concluded that the mutually reinforcing interaction between the empathic caregiver and the infant enables the infant to develop internal supply lines of pleasure. These reciprocal sources of pleasure, deriving from empathic care, are detailed in Table 9.2. In his book *Early Deprivation of Empathic Care* Weil hypothesizes that "an infant's chronic deprivation of empathic care amounts to the infant's chronic loss of these supply lines of pleasure" (p. 43) and that unempathic care leads to a mutually reinforcing pattern of

TABLE 9.2. Supply Lines of Infant Pleasure

The caregiver's persisting visual, auditory, and tactile contacts with the infant as a source for pleasurable attention

The mutual pleasure-resonance between caregiver and infant as a source of pleasure

The caregiver's tenderness as a basis for pleasure

The caregiver's resonant tuning in to the infant's distress as a basis for protection, comforting, and pleasure

---

Note. Adapted with permission from Weil (1992). Copyright 1992 by International Universities Press, Inc.

interaction leading to reciprocal angry distress in both the infant and the caregiver.

Weil found that in the majority of cases chronic deprivation of empathic care in infancy leads not only to chronic loss of pleasure but also to the formation of relatively fixed patterns of hyper- and hypoarousal states in the infants. Table 9.3 summarizes these states.

These patterns of hyper- and hypoarousal during infancy are pervasive and persistent, and Weil hypothesizes that they correspond to the diffuse psychophysiological regulatory system "of the brain and its ascending and descending irradiations from the base of the brain up to the cerebral cortex as well as down to the total body musculature" (pp. 56–57). The effect of chronic loss of "supply lines of pleasure" may have other physiological manifestations, as the research by Heath (Heath, 1964; Heath and Gallant, 1964) on the brain's hedonic control centers in the limbic–hypothalamic–reticular areas suggests. Weil documents findings similar to his of pathological hyperactivity and hypoactivity resulting from early disturbance in mother–infant interaction, namely, those by Bender (1935), Goldfarb (1943), Langmeier and Matejcek (1975), Money (1980), Ribble (1965), Robertson (1962), and Spitz (1951). Weil also cites Greenspan (1981, 1987, 1989, 1992), whose studies reached similar conclusions about the sequelae of disturbance in the archaic relatedness of infant and mother, finding diffuse and persistent

TABLE 9.3. Hyper and Hypo States of Behavior

Hyper	Hyper states of consciousness and wakefulness; exaggerated amounts of random activity and increased speed of activity; repetitive, rhythmic behavior such as rocking, thumb sucking, masturbation, and headrolling; exaggerated sensitivity and reactivity to stimuli; muscular tension, stiffness, rigidity, and exaggerated intensity of muscular force; exaggerated visceral activities including pulse, rate of respiration, speed of eating, and frequency of urination and defecation.
Hypo	Hypo states of consciousness, including lethargy and somnolence; reduced quantity of movement and speed; reduced sensitivity to stimuli; muscular flaccidity and reduced muscular force; and reduced visceral activity including lowered heart rate and reduced rate of respiration, speed of eating, and frequency of urination and defecation.

Note. Adapted with permission from Weil (1992). Copyright 1992 by International Universities Press, Inc.

TABLE 9.4. Greenspan's Model of Ego Development with Superimposed Effects of Early Deprivation: Maladaptive Hyperactivity/Hypoactivity, Distress, and Loss of Pleasure

Infant age	Normoactivity (adaptive)	Hyperactivity (maladaptive)	Hypoactivity (maladaptive)
0–3 months	Relaxed. Sleeps at regular times; cries only occasionally. Alert; returns gaze when spoken to; brightens up when rocked, touched, or otherwise stimulated.	Rigid. Becomes completely distracted by any sights, noises, touch, movement. Often upset and crying.	Does not respond to stimuli. Sleeps most of the day. Shows little interest in anything or anyone.
2–7 months	Very interested in people, especially parents. Looks, smiles, responds to their voices and touch with signs of pleasure.	Demands for tranquilizing contacts. Insists on being held all the time. Will not sleep without being held.	Withdrawn. Uninterested in mother, father, or other primary caregivers. Usually looks *away from* rather than *at* people.
3–10 months	Interacts purposefully. Smiles in response to a smile. Able to get involved with toys. Shows pleasure when interacting with a person.	Demands constant interaction. Displays temper tantrums or withdrawal if caretaker does not respond to its signals.	Unresponsive. Seems oblivious to caregivers. Does not respond to their smiles, voices, or attempts at interaction.
9–24 months	Manifests a wide range of socially meaningful behavior and feelings. Plays and interacts with parents. Able to go from interaction to separation and reunion with organized affects, including pleasure. Can explore new objects and new people.	Behavior and affect completely random and chaotic. Toddler almost always appears "out of control," with aggressive affects predominating.	Compliant. Rarely initiates behavior. Mostly passive and withdrawn.

Note. Adapted with permission from Weil (1992). Copyright 1992 by International Universities Press, Inc.

patterns of hyperactivity and hypoactivity, and are summarized in
Table 9.4.

It should be noted that Weil does not dismiss the genetic and
organic determinants of hyper- and hypoactivity in infants but
advocates an interactive model of development in which innate
biological endowment both shapes and is shaped by the infant's lived
experience. He cites numerous research studies that support the
conclusion that infantile stress produced by dynamic environmental
influences produces prolonged alterations in central nervous system
metabolism involving multiple neurotransmitters.

Weil hypothesizes that hyper- and hypoactive behavior in infants is not merely pathological but also has an adaptive function
whose purpose is to restore the supply lines of pleasure through
compensatory processes. For example, the disturbed infant's intense
motor agitation and constant crying may ultimately force the inat-
tentive parent to respond to its needs. Alternately, the deprived
infant's head banging and rocking may provide for itself the sensory
stimulation missing from its pre-object relatedness with its primary
caregiver. This self-stimulation may be focused on areas of the body
with erotic potential in order to provide a source of the missing
pleasurable interaction with the primary caregiver. Weil cites
Ainsworth's research (Ainsworth et al., 1978a, b) as best describing
the means by which early deficits or disturbance in maternal care
lead to the establishment of two general forms of pathological
attachment. Weil also describes four types of compensatory supply
lines of pleasure, summarized in Table 9.5.

PATHOLOGY OF THE BIPERSONAL FIELD

Once internalized, the successes and failures of pre-object development persist into adulthood. If pathology once structured the interaction between mother and infant, it similarly will structure
intrapsychic personality development and will become manifest in
the interaction between patient and therapist in the psychotherapeutic and psychoanalytic situations. Psychotherapy takes place
between the subjectivities of both patient and therapist, subjectivities that have been shaped by developmental realities, both adaptive
and pathological (Stolorow, 1991; Stolorow, Brandchaft, and Atwood,
1987). In this regard, Robert Langs's (1976, 1978a, b) descriptions

TABLE 9.5. Compensatory Supply Lines of Pleasure

Type	Activity level	Compensatory activities
A	Hyper	Crying may become a way for the deprived infant to gain contact, attention, and pleasurable care from a withdrawn or indifferent caregiver.
B	Hyper	The infant may turn away from contacts with its depriving caregiver and turn toward its own rudimentary ego motor manipulation of the inanimate environment.
C	Hyper	The infant may turn away from contacts with its depriving caregiver and turn toward sensory contacts with its own body surface, body products, and body orifices, and to sensation seeking associated with one or more of the five senses.
D	Hypo	The infant may turn away from physical or emotional contacts with its depriving caregiver and withdraw into states of lethargy and sleep.

Note. Adapted with permission from Weil (1992). Copyright 1992 by International Universities Press, Inc.

of communicative pathology between patient and psychotherapist are of considerable interest.

Langs described the psychotherapeutic and psychoanalytic situations as interactional in their essence, calling them a "bipersonal field," a term first coined by the Barangers (Baranger and Baranger, 1966). According to Langs, each communication within the field receives input from both patient and therapist along an interactional interface. The field has a framework: the ground rules of the psychotherapeutic situation. Communications relate either to the manifest content, which is in itself without dynamic meaning, or to "derivative communications," which may have dynamic content.

Langs stated that there are two types of derivative communications. Type One derivatives are inferences about unconscious processes that are derived from the manifest content. For example, if the patient reports a frightening dream about exploring a dangerous, dark cave containing poisonous snakes, the therapist may surmise that the dream relates to some associated sexual conflict, although in the absence of any overt or disguised allusions to actual sexual concerns such an inference is not sufficient evidence on which to base a definitive interpretation. Now if the patient, after telling us the dream, goes on to say that he had difficulty maintaining an erection during sexual intercourse with his wife the day before, shortly after feeling jealous of his wife's relationship with her male supervisor, and that during sex he had a fleeting, exciting impulse to hurt her, such an association contributes to a vastly more definitive and dynamic understanding of the patient's symptom of impotence and the latent meaning of his dream. Langs referred to such inferences as Type Two derivatives. Type Two derivatives are, by their nature, organized around specific "adaptive contexts" and lend themselves to the formulation of interventions and interpretations based on an accurate and empathic understanding of the patient's unconscious meaning. According to Langs, the optimal bipersonal field is characterized by a secure framework, symbolic expression, and Type Two derivatives. This is the ideal of the psychoanalytic situation. Langs called such a field a Type A field.

Langs differentiates two other fields, the Type B and Type C fields, which have primarily pathological significance. The Type B field is characterized by projective identification and enactment. In a Type B field the ground rules of the treatment are altered in crucial ways. Speech is employed primarily for its discharge qualities rather than its communicative qualities. Because the psychotherapeutic situation is fundamentally interactional, the source of such discharge activities may be the patient or the therapist, or both. In contrast, one or both participants of the Type C field eradicate, through both action and language, communications that link them. Symbolic expression is significantly impaired, and speech becomes concrete in its implications, omitting even disguised references to specific adaptive contexts. According to Langs, the purpose of the Type C field is the creation of an impenetrable barrier to deep emotional communication; to this end, speech is denuded of communicative meaning. Langs called the creation of such an alienated form of relatedness a type of "negative projective identification."

While Langs did not take developmental influences into consideration in this study, I believe one may readily note that the two types of interactional pathology he described are similar to the two types of pathology noted in the observations of infants and mothers by Ainsworth, Gaddini, Weil, and Greenspan. What Langs described as a Type B field, which is characterized by action discharge and projective identification by one or both participants, is similar to (1) Gaddini's concept of a borderline environment characterized by maternal ambivalence, three-month colic, and early psychosomatic responses (with later development of language difficulties and the physical expression of symbolic meanings); (2) Ainsworth's concept of Group C ambivalently attached babies, who alternated anxiously between avoidance and clinging in response to unpredictable parental support; and (3) Weil's concept of hyper states of behavior and (4) Greenspan's concept of maladaptive hyperactivity, both of which evolve in response to early difficulties in parental care. Langs's Type C field, in which communication is deprived of anything more than superficial meaning, is similar to (1) Gaddini's concept of a pathogenic environment, characterized by maternal unavailability, lack of reciprocity, infant apathy, and distance from the mother and later by nonrelatedness, lack of playfulness, and symbolic disturbance; (2) Ainsworth's concept of Type A avoidantly attached babies, who are impassive, withdrawn, and gravitate to the nonhuman environment in response to their mother's aversion to physical and emotional contact or to the direct expression of her hostility; and (3) Weil's concept of hypo states of behavior and (4) Greenspan's concept of maladaptive hypoactivity, both of which are manifestations of exhaustion from efforts to engage the primary caregiver in pleasurable interaction. Finally, Langs's Type A field, in which both participants are engaging in attuned and meaningful communication in depth, is similar to (1) Gaddini's description of the facilitating environment, (2) Ainsworth's description of Type B securely attached babies, (3) Weil's description of empathic care, and (4) Greenspan's description of adaptive normoactivity.

The implication of these similarities is to draw together the work of a wide variety of researchers. The studies of pioneers in ego psychology, object relations theory, self psychology, attachment theory, and infant research show striking similarities in their descriptions of the nature, process, and outcome of the competency, partial disturbance, or failure of pre-object development. Such a stance also enables one to note the similarities, rather than the differences, between Freud's theory of signal anxiety and subsequent descriptions of projective and introjective identification and transmuting internalization (as I discussed in Chapter Three). Such views bear directly on the observational studies described in this chapter. For example, what might the correlation be between Kleinian descriptions of the manic defense and Weil's descriptions of hyper states, or between Fairbairn's and Klein's descriptions of a paranoid-schizoid stance and avoidant attachment? What might the correlation be between pathological projective identification as described by Bion and the tendency of babies in disturbed dyads to attack their mother's body? What is the correlation between Kohut's descriptions of self-fragmentation in response to empathic failure and descriptions by attachment theorists of insecure attachment secondary to destructive parental behavior? What is the correlation between Winnicott's descriptions of a false self that provides precocious self-caring capacities and Bergman and Escalona's (1949) descriptions of precocious ego development? If we, as observers of human development, attempt to suspend the usual polemics concerning the differences between our various theoretical viewpoints, we may be able to increasingly discern an emerging cohesiveness of opinion and singularity of purpose.

The actualities of the psychoanalytic and psychotherapeutic situations provide the patient with numerous occasions for experiencing both emotional closeness and distance within the boundaries of the treatment relationship. This is so because of the relative frequency of appointments contrasted with the relative abstinence and limits of analytic technique, the intimacy and depth of personal revelation contrasted with the relative anonymity of the analyst, and so on. The patient experiences the analyst as both a familiar ally and an unknown intruder, as both a mentor who prompts emotional growth through the empathic provision of insight-promoting relatedness and an unempathic caregiver who deprives the self of vital emotional supplies. The psychoanalytic situation promotes attachment through the reliability of its setting, the frequency of meetings, its persistence over time, and the empathic interpretative activity of the analyst, which promotes intimacy and a sense of emotional proximity. But the psychoanalytic situation also promotes an anxiety analogous to the eight-month-old's displeasure at the approach of an unfamiliar person (Spitz, 1959), because the analyst is out of sight behind the couch, is abstinent according to psychoanalytic technique, maintains the formalism of the ground rules of the treatment situation, and occasionally misunderstands the meaning of the patient's communications and reenacts any traumatic failures of empathic care that characterized the patient's pre-object relatedness. Such potentially painful eventualities of the psychoanalytic situation are indications not of faultiness in its design but, rather, of its unique capacity for eliciting reenactments of the original successes and failures of childhood development that date back even to pre-object experiences. These reenactments inevitably pattern the transference and countertransference and provide the opportunity for the mediation of the patient's infantile traumatic state in the analytic situation.

CHAPTER TEN

Ambivalent Relatedness
and Avoidant Relatedness

I N THIS CHAPTER I elaborate a hypothesis of pathology of signal affects based on two forms of disturbed pre-object relatedness. These disturbances result from impairment of infant–caregiver interaction. I originally derived the hypothesis reconstructively from my work with adult patients. The plausibility of the hypothesis was then subsequently supported by direct experience of its clinical utility and by my discovery of the research of Ainsworth, R. Gaddini, Weil, and Greenspan on early pathology of affect regulation and attachment behavior. Their descriptions substantiate the inference that pre-object internalization of pathology in the infant–mother dyad is etiological in this type of pathological development.

There is, in my view, strong correspondence between what Ainsworth described as Group C ambivalently attached infants and a type of internal pathology of affect regulation I regularly encounter in adult patients. I will call this form of pathology, after Ainsworth, ambivalent relatedness. Here, the internal part of the self that receives signal affects is inconsistent in its response, effectively muting the danger signal with suitable defenses at times but failing to respond effectively at other times. There is an internal turbulence in the individual's capacity to respond to his or her own affect signals.

Excerpts from this chapter were presented, under different titles, to the 34th Winter Meeting of the American Academy of Psychoanalysis, December 1990; the Vancouver Psychoanalytic Psychotherapy Society, February 1991; the Seattle Psychoanalytic Society, March 1991; and the Northwest Alliance for Psychoanalytic Study, June 1991.

Such inconstancy of internal affect regulation results from internalization of an inconsistent or chaotic interactional regulatory system formed by the infant and its primary caregiver, a system that begins in earliest pre-object development and then subsequently congeals in the baby's emerging character and way of relating to objects. Thus, lack of "goodness of fit" between the infant and mother leads to ambivalence in both mother and baby, resulting in a deepening cycle of inconstant signaling and receiving and endless affect turbulence, a cycle that becomes internalized as an inconstant way of responding to one's self and others.

Similar correspondence also exists between Ainsworth's Group A avoidantly attached infants and those adults whose internal pre-object state is what I will call avoidant relatedness. Avoidant relatedness is characterized by sign negation. Adults whose affect regulation functions in this way do not recognize or respond to their own affect signals. They are detached, unemotional, concrete, and existentially absent in the core of their self-experience.

Studies that follow the results of attachment disturbances in infancy into later infancy and childhood are currently emerging. Osofsky (1987) reported how the infants of detached, unemotional mothers begin to themselves appear detached, bland, and avoidant by six months of age, implying that the babies' internalization of the pre-object infant–mother bond creates lasting distortions in their affect-regulating and object-relating capacities. Fonagy, Steele, Moran, Steele, and Higgitt (1993) demonstrated how the security of an infant's relationship with both parents at 12 and 18 months can be predicted prior to birth on the basis of qualitative aspects of the parents' accounts of their own childhoods on a structured interview.[1] Bowlby (1989) described the persistence of symptomatology resulting from insecure attachment in infancy on follow-up during the first five years. A feedback loop is implied: Insecurely attached babies must certainly be more difficult and less rewarding to care for and thus are less likely to elicit attuned caregiving. Vicious cycles and asynchronies must certainly develop in which pre-object disturbances in maternal attunement lead eventually to insecure attachment, dis-

---

[1]The interview tool used was the Adult Attachment Interview, first developed by Mary Main and her coworkers (Main et al., 1985). With the creation of this instrument, the authors introduced to attachment theory an emphasis on the *subjective representation* of attachment experiences as central to the emergence of subsequent pathology.

turbed affect signaling, and pathological object relating, all of which lead to further disturbances in the mother's capacity to respond effectively to her baby. This is not an entirely hopeless situation, however: Bowlby noted that improved attunement to signaled distress leads to a reduction in the observed distress, and Lamb (1987) showed that disturbance in infant attachment patterns does not invariably lead to later pathology of attachment relationships. It is intriguing to speculate that adults with one of the kinds of psychopathology described in this chapter may be suffering from sequelae of the very early relational difficulties first categorized by Ainsworth. Long-term follow-up studies would clarify this relationship.

PATHOLOGY OF SIGNAL AFFECTS

Signal anxiety and signal affects are the result of the interaction of an innate developmental process with the relative success or failure of infant–mother affective interchange. Adult signal affects derive from the internalization of the affect-regulating successes and failures of the infant–mother pair beginning even prior to the infant's differentiation of self-representation from object representation. As a result, signaling aspects of the ego derive from what was originally the baby in the pair, and receiving functions of the ego derive from what was originally the mother-experienced-as-auxiliary-ego-by-the-baby. Receiver functions of the ego determine later capacities for affect regulation and defense. These functions develop in part through innate developmental givens and in part through primary identification. Where the mother's response is not adequate to promote quiescence, the infant's sign of distress is not extinguished. Table 10.1 correlates the regulation of signal affects described in this chapter with the forms of behavioral health and disturbance described in the previous chapter.

According to Segal (in press), all aspects of the self require external facilitation in order to develop, even pathological aspects: Just as narcissistic health requires selfobject support originating in parental empathy, so too does narcissistic disturbance evolve from a matrix of pathogenic selfobject support for the emerging pathology. Once this situation becomes internalized, the response of the ego will not be adequate to recognize affects as signals or to establish sufficiently adaptive defenses against unpleasurable thoughts, wishes, perceptions, and feelings. In other words, psychopathology results from a signal affect that cannot adequately be received.

The etiology of psychopathology is often complex and cannot be understood in a simplistic way. For example, the infant may suffer an inborn anatomic or biochemical brain dysfunction that disturbs its capacity to process, experience, and regulate affect. Or the nature of the baby's distress is not amenable to extinction despite good-enough caretaking, as in, for example, excruciating pain from chronic illness that can be mitigated but not fully soothed by any quality or amount of holding. Or an internal disturbance may alter the infant's perception of the mother, distorting her capacity to respond adequately to need; such internal disturbance may lead to disturbances in the actual interaction with the mother, which may then exacerbate the innate disturbance. Or the mother's actual capacity for good-enough attunement may be temporarily impaired, disturbed, or limited because of family crisis, depression, or narcissistic injury, impairing her ability to respond adequately to the child's needs at a developmentally sensitive juncture. These examples are merely suggestive of the variety and scope of sources for the ultimate development of disturbances in receiver functioning of the ego. However, once disturbed, the impairment of gamma-function leads to an inability to link together sense impressions and affect, psyche and soma, self and object.

Thus, the nature of the causes for an individual's relative incapacity to adequately receive, tolerate, neutralize, and regulate signal affects becomes an obvious and crucial question, both as it applies to

TABLE 10.1. Terminology Used by Various Researchers to Describe the Result of the Caregiver's Response to the Distress Sign

	Sign extinction	Sign turbulence	Sign negation
Ainsworth	Secure attachment	Ambivalent attachment	Avoidant attachment
R. Gaddini	Facilitating	Borderline	Pathogenic
Weil	Empathic care	Hyper states	Hypo states
Greenspan	Adaptive normoactivity	Maladaptive hyperactivity	Maladaptive hypoactivity
Langs	Type A field	Type B field	Type C field

the external interpersonal relationships of self to object as well as to the internalized pre-object relationship, that is, the intrapersonal relationship between an affect-signaling and an affect-regulating part of the self. In order to demonstrate the application of this way of understanding internal conflict, I will describe in terms of their consequences for the development of signal affects the two forms of behavioral pathology originating in the pre-object relatedness of infant and mother.

AMBIVALENT RELATEDNESS

In the pre-object state of ambivalent relatedness the original affect that is signaled is itself considered to be dangerous by the mother, who responds with a signal affect of her own. Since the mother in the pre-object state is not experienced as differentiated clearly from one's self (although from an objective vantage point the receiver might actually have been the mother who was holding the infant), such an experience creates two parts of the self that cannot communicate adequately with one another because each part feels overwhelmed and unassisted by the signaled other. When internalized, such a situation would seem to serve as a forerunner of emotional conflict and pathological defense.

Repeated experience in which the infant cannot elicit a soothing response from the external environment leads to an internal situation in which there is a disturbance in the mental or emotional receiver for the communicated danger signal. In such a situation there are two signalers in internal reality, corresponding to the infant and the mother in external reality, each of whom attempts unsuccessfully to signal the other partner as receiver of an impending trauma. The relationship is inherently pathological because the confluence of opposing danger signals and the absence of an ego state capable of effectively receiving the projected affect creates sign turbulence rather than sign extinction. Infant research has substantiated the view that when the caretaker's response is not sufficient to allay the distress of the infant, the intensity of the affect content of the infant's response may become heightened (Brazelton, 1969; Brazelton and Als, 1979; Brazelton and Cramer, 1990; Emde, 1983, 1984; 1988a, b; Emde, Gaensbauer, and Harmon, 1976; Spitz, 1965; Stern, 1985a). In the psychoanalytic situation such patients are prone to respond with panic states, externalizing defenses, acting out, defensive and adaptive sexualization, and intense ambivalence. The following vignette describes the way in which such pathology of affect regulation sometimes enters the psychoanalytic therapy of adults.

A middle-aged male entered treatment after a long history of chronic depression treated unsuccessfully by past psychiatrists with antidepressant medication and supportive psychotherapy. The man had been married four times, each marriage ending after a short period of time in divorce. He had been unfaithful during each of his marriages and had been sexually promiscuous since. He had a talent for seducing women. He took little pleasure in this because he instantly lost all interest in the women as people as soon as he reached climax. He felt he was missing out on something crucial in life and yearned for a meaningful relationship. He described underachievement in his current job because of difficulty learning new tasks, and he related this to the "dyslexia" he suffered from in elementary school. He had many painful memories of being unable to learn simple concepts as a child because of constant mental confusion.

At the beginning of therapy the patient would frequently yawn while talking during sessions and would rub his eyes as though about to fall asleep. The early part of his therapy enabled him to become more aware of his hostility toward me, which he was attempting to both express and conceal through boredom, sleepiness, and mental distraction in the sessions. When we attempted to explore why he might choose to express his aggression in this particular form he remembered a childhood symptom: He had severe insomnia from age four to eight and would spend every night sleepwalking from bed to bed among his brothers. He realized that he had gone from bed to bed as a child and from marriage to marriage as an adult. He would awaken in bed with one brother and not know how he had gotten there, finally fall asleep again and later awaken in another brother's bed.

The next year was spent trying to reconstruct the reason for this childhood sleepwalking, which I surmised was an attempt to avoid awareness of some trauma that was disturbing the child during the night. Gradually, the patient became able to relate this to memories of his mother's sexual promiscuity throughout his childhood. His father was frequently away from home because of the nature of his work, and his mother had a succession of strange men in the house during the night. Furthermore, she had impeded her son's capacity to be aware of what was happening by denying the validity of his perceptions. For example, one night he had seen a strange man walking nude down the hallway from his mother's bedroom to use the bathroom. When he asked his mother the following morning who the man was, his mother responded sharply, "There was no man here. You must have been dreaming." This response created doubt in her son's mind as to whether he had been awake or asleep.

The patient identified both with his mother's promiscuity and with his family's secrecy about the infidelity. His internalization of his mother's (and father's) denial about the hateful sexuality that pervaded his home led to a learning inhibition. To learn was to know what he was forbidden to know; therefore, the patient restricted his own ability to learn. His childhood insomnia was related to distressing knowledge about what was transpiring in his mother's bed. He went from bed to bed to avoid this knowledge and to identify with his mother. It now became clearer that my earlier interpretation of the meaning of his eye rubbing was incomplete. The eye rubbing in his analytic sessions not only expressed and denied his hostility but was also a way to deny to himself what he saw with his own two eyes as well as an indication of the somnolence and withdrawal that threatened to intervene as a further defense, adaptation, and compensation. The patient was unable to fully receive what he knew and had to disavow the significance of his own signals of distress to himself.

Another example of ambivalent relatedness comes from Ogden's (1989a) paper on what he calls the "autistic–contiguous position." Ogden, expanding on the ideas of Bick (1968) and Tustin (1980, 1984, 1986), conceived of this position as the earliest state of mental and emotional development, a state during which nascent self-experience coalesces around sensory experience at the skin surface. The self coheres around the sensation of the skin touching hard objects or soft amorphous shapes. These contact boundaries are employed concretely for the purpose of self-definition. Ogden (1989a) cites the following case of a 25-year-old graduate student who was terrified of the fog and of going crazy.

Ms. K's mother contracted spinal meningitis when the patient was four months old and was hospitalized for fourteen months. From the time that the patient's mother returned home, Mrs. K was confined to a wheelchair and tyrannically ruled the house from her metal chair. The patient's earliest memory (which seemed to her as much like a dream as a memory) was of reaching out to her mother in her wheelchair and being pushed away by her mother. At the same moment, the patient, in this memory, looked out of the window and saw a small child falling through the ice on the pond that was located just behind the patient's house. Mrs. K said, "You'd better go save her."

Expanding on Ogden's ensuing discussion, I would interpret the patient's screen memory of a child falling through the ice as symbolizing a part of the patient's self signaling desperately for help. This aspect of her ego feels that her mother could not adequately receive her communicated affect signal and feels that, although she reached out to her mother, her mother pushed away any awareness of her distress. Because of the loss of the affect-regulating functions her mother might have provided, a panic state ensues in which she senses the collapse of her underlying ego support. In Ogden's words, she "falls through the containing surface of self (initially created in the interaction of mother and infant)" (p. 134). The mother in this "memory" not only relates to Ms. K's relationship with her actual mother but also symbolizes a deficient aspect of her ability to understand or contain her own emotional distress. Ms. K anxiously confuses feelings with "drowning" in panic, represented by the countersignaling behavior of the intended receiver. In this scenario the older child who must save the drowning child symbolizes that aspect of the patient's ego which must adapt to the deficiencies of the receiver and "take care of herself," adapting as best she can to her own unabsorbed panic state.

AVOIDANT RELATEDNESS

Another cause for the relative incapacity to receive communicated signal affects may be the decathexis of the signaler by the receiver, that is, a pre-object state of avoidant relatedness. Furman and Furman (1984) described a phenomenon of unconscious, intermit-

tent, sudden, and almost complete withdrawal of emotional investment in one's child—in other words, abruptly treating the child as
though he or she were nonexistent—which they observed in the
mothers of certain of their pediatric patients and traced in their
adult analysands. They cited an emotionally painful anecdote of a
latency-age patient with severe ego disturbances who was described
by his teachers as frequently acting as though he were on "cloud
nine." He would stand very close to the analyst during his appointments, take the analyst's head in his hands, and turn his head so
that they were talking eye to eye at an intrusively close range. No
understanding of this perplexing behavior sufficed until the child's
father was questioned. He immediately understood its source and
explained that unless his wife looked directly at the person she was
talking to, that person could never be certain his wife was paying
any attention to him or her. He said, "If I want to ask her something
or tell her something and she is, for example, reading the paper, I
go and take the paper out of her hands and sit in front of her to talk.
If I don't do this, she will respond as if she had listened to me, but
it will soon turn out she had not heard a word I said" (p. 423). When
the Furmans spoke with the mother about this behavior, she confirmed it and related a time when the child was 18 months old and
she was giving a large dinner party on behalf of some friends for
many people she did not know.

> About 10:00 p.m. the doorbell rang and she opened the door to be
> greeted by a stranger she assumed was yet another of her guests she
> did not know. It took her some moments to understand what he was
> trying to tell her. He was explaining that he had found a toddler in
> pajamas wandering the sidewalk in front of her house. He had been
> driving by and had stopped to try to help the child, and was wondering
> if she knew where the boy lived. Only at this point did she see the child
> whose hand the man held. "Would you believe that at first I did not
> even recognize my own son? I was so absorbed in the party, I just did
> not see or recognize him." (p. 423)

The Furmans pointed out that this particular mother was not
depressed, and they distinguished the intermittent decathexis by
this parent from the emotional withdrawal of a depressed parent
who might remain fully invested in his or her child despite being
depressed. They also distinguished intermittent decathexis from a
defensive or angry withdrawal, as in giving the other person the cold

shoulder, which they show is conscious, only partially decathects the other, and is associated with emotional pain. The "cold shoulder" is a "simulated decathexis," unlike the actual process they described in which the parent's withdrawal of emotional investment in the child is unconscious, sudden, and almost complete.

Tronick, Als, Adamson, Wise, and Brazelton (1978, cited in Tyson and Tyson, 1990) conducted an experiment that applies indirectly to the Furmans' observations. In their experimental setup the mother and her infant are facing each other, and the mother is instructed not to respond as she normally would to her baby. She is told not to look directly into the infant's eyes but to look above the baby's head while remaining physically still and emotionally impassive. The infants in this study responded to this experimentally induced decathexis dramatically. Tyson and Tyson (1990) described the infant's reaction as follows:

> First the infant tries to recapture the mother's gaze visually by looking around corners, moving his eyes from side to side, moving his head back and forward, in clear attempts to reestablish visual interaction. Before long the infant becomes distressed and reaches out for contact with the mother using his arms, legs, and body, as well as leaning forward with his head. Finally the infant gives up, his posture collapses, and he withdraws. This is soon followed by renewed attempts to contact the nonreciprocating, blank-faced, distant mother. Following the experiment the mother reengages herself with her infant, and very shortly they are able to regain their communication. (p. 124)

Given the near-catastrophic reaction to a single episode of experimentally induced decathexis, one can easily imagine the ongoing effects of the cumulative trauma of repeated unpredictable episodes of intermittent decathexis throughout development. The Furmans demonstrated how the frequent withdrawals by the latency-age boy, similar to the withdrawal response of the infants in the Tronick experiment, represented both an identification with his mother and a defensive turning of passive into active. Put another way, the child decathected others as his mother decathected him. But, more pertinent to the subject of this chapter, the Furmans showed how the child had internalized his mother's behavior *as an attitude toward himself*, demonstrated by his "inability to keep himself safe—he endured many accidents and self-injuries—and . . . [by his] inability consistently to cathect his various ego functions"

(p. 424). I speculate that once children have internalized their caretaker's intermittent inability to cathect their signal, they cannot adequately cathect the signaler function of their own ego; their affect sign is blocked from achieving symbolic representation by the negative receiving function of their own ego, leading to sign negation. Sign negation is a pathological process that is not to be confused with sign extinction, which results from the caregiver's normally adaptive response to the infant's distress. In sign negation the communicated sign of distress is not attended by the receiver; it is negated, canceled, rendered meaningless.[2] Sign negation is also to be distinguished from sign turbulence, a situation in which the infant's signal affect causes distress in the caretaker. However, the very presence of the caretaker's distress ensures that the infant's sign is given meaning, albeit an idiosyncratic and pathological meaning. Sign negation leads to a negation of the signaler aspect of the ego and thus a negation of any developing representation relating to the signal affect or the self that experiences it.

When the communicated affect is not received as a danger signal because it has been decathected or rendered nonexistent or meaningless, a state of mental confusion, of being emotionally lost, ensues. This is followed by diffuse panic and ultimately by helpless emotional withdrawal. According to the Furmans, being treated as nonexistent creates major developmental difficulties that compound throughout life. Narcissistic injury to the developing child results in a number of ego disturbances, including the inability to cathect the self-representation enough to take sufficient care of one's self, difficulty in forming an integrated body image, poor self-esteem regulation, and lasting narcissistic rage. Later, the internalized ego disturbances interfere with the development of considerate relationships with others. The fear of being decathected leads to profound separation anxiety, which creates havoc with the age-appropriate relinquishment of earlier modes of relationship, as during toilet training, the entry into school situations, the development of peer relationships

---

[2]One additional metaphor that might describe the operation of sign negation is a current technique for sound muffling used in noisy industrial environments: A computer monitors and samples repetitive mechanical sounds in the workplace and instantly generates and then transmits through a loudspeaker a waveform that is identical to the offending noise but 180° out of phase with it, thus canceling the sound. This method is now being tested as an "electronic muffler" for automobiles. Whether sign negation operates by countercathexis, decathexis, or some other pathway is a topic for further study.

during the latency years, and during the object removal of adolescence.

Ogden (1979) described the unconscious fear of being decathected, a fear that renders an individual vulnerable to complicity with the projective identifications of others:

> [There exists] a pressure on an infant to behave in a manner congruent with the mother's pathology and the ever-present threat that if the infant were to fail to comply, he would become non-existent for the mother. This threat is the "muscle" behind the demand for compliance: "If you are not what I need you to be, you don't exist for me," or in other language, "I can only see in you what I put there, and so if I don't see that in you, I see nothing." (p. 360)

These disturbances in the caregiver lead a child to internalize a deficient receiver function during the pre-object stages of development. The internalization of this pathological ego function results in the negation of the signaler aspect of the ego and of the danger affects it signals. This now internalized aspect of the ego intermittently decathects the self-representation whenever it makes demands on it for self-care. As I understand them, sign negation and sign turbulence are not necessarily the sole result of a developmental arrest or of a deficiency in what an individual phase-appropriately needs for ego maturation. These defects are a result of an internalization of a pathological relational process. The individual suffers not merely from a deficit but from a disturbance of the infant–mother dyad that a part of the ego has internalized. Furthermore, the pathological process that has been internalized may itself produce mental, emotional, and physiological deficits for which the individual must compensate. The difference between sign turbulence and sign negation could be likened to the difference between a child suffering from chronic malnutrition and a child suffering from chronic food poisoning.

Decathected individuals cannot regulate their own affects, cannot receive their own signals of danger, and unconsciously treat the distressed parts of themselves as nonexistent. Meanwhile, they may simultaneously and chaotically increase the urgency and drama of any communicated signal affects in order to force the receiver to pay attention, to desperately coerce cathexis of themselves by the receiver. Weil (1992) described the potentially adaptive effect of behavioral hyperactivity as a compensatory means of securing sources

of pleasure. Similarly, the Furmans described how children sub-
jected to intermittent decathexis may resort to affect storms in order
to capture their mother's attention. Krystal (1988) noted how adult
patients with disturbance in affect tolerance can generate regressive chaotic emotional outbursts in hopes of coercing a caretaking
response from those to whom they are attached. Pathological disturbance in the mother's capacity to receive and mediate the infant's
distress leads (via intermodal exchange) to a defective capacity in
the infant's ego to receive its own affect signals and to generate an
adaptive response.

A young father consulted me in a depressive crisis. He had
severe doubts about consulting an analyst, as people close to
him had had bad experiences with analysts. Nevertheless, he
felt he had nowhere else to turn. During the second appointment he described his conflicted relationship with his oldest
son. His son had been born during a troubled time in his
marriage. As a result, he never felt as attached to this child as
to his other children. He made great efforts to be a good parent,
and, indeed, the boy did not seem to be suffering from this secret
emotional conflict of his father. They got along well together,
and the boy seemed to be developing normally for a boy his age.
Still, the man always thought of this child as his "adopted son."
      At one point in the second session the patient suddenly
looked over to me and asked, "Do you understand what I mean?"
I answered that it was clear that an answer to his question was
very important to him and that while it would be a simple
matter for me to answer his question, I wondered if more could
be learned by paying attention to why he had suddenly felt the
urgency to have an answer to this particular question at this
particular time.
      While the patient was clearly annoyed by my not answering
directly, he immediately recalled that when his son was a year
old, he told his wife about his conflict and she "had not been able
to understand" why he felt the way he did. This was terribly
painful to him, and he feared that I, like his wife, would not be
able to understand him.
      But I also wondered if the patient himself understood how
he felt, and I asked him. He gave me a curious look and said,
"You know, I *don't* understand myself. These feelings seem
incomprehensible to me." He said he realized that these feelings

of not being able to understand himself came before his wife's failure to understand him (Thus, in a sense her failure to understand intensified a preexisting emotion). He didn't know where this feeling came from, but he sensed it had been there a long time.

The patient began the third appointment by recalling these remarks and spontaneously volunteered that he thought his problem might have something to do with his relationship with his mother. He said that for as long as he could remember, he felt his mother was indifferent to his troubles. One of his earliest memories was of running down the hallway at full speed and banging his head on the wall, thinking that if he hurt himself enough he would get his mother to attend to him. Indeed, this did have the desired effect.

I said that he was concerned not only that analysis would be futile, like hitting his head against the wall, but also that the only way he could make me understand him would be to be hurtful to himself.

He smiled and said that he *had* had the fantasy of wanting to be unconscious so as not to feel the intense emotional pain he was in. But my remark had made him remember something else, namely, that part of the fantasy had been that he would render himself unconscious by hitting his head against the wall. He now told me that he suffered from colitis and wondered if he might also be "hitting his guts against the wall."

Later I learned that the patient's mother had been adopted, had suffered a sequence of profound losses during her childhood, and had been under severe stress during her pregnancy with the patient. During infancy the patient had chronic diarrhea and was hospitalized for a month; after he returned home, the diarrhea continued. He was diagnosed as having "failure to thrive" until he was 18 months old.

This patient's asking me if I understood him was his way of signaling an internal danger to me. My calling his attention to the danger his question signaled to a part of himself seemed to open up the whole subject of his pre-object relations. At this level it was not conflict between intact intrapsychic structures that was being signaled but the imminence of an internal catastrophe related to the interruption of an affect-regulating prestructure. The current colitis resulted from the same disturbances in the pre-object functioning of his body ego that had led to his infantile diarrhea. His agitated depression was related to a difficulty in clearly differentiating his internalized object's (and originally his mother's) anxiety and lack of understanding from his own. He now inflicted panic and pain upon himself in order to attract sufficient understanding not only from the environment but also from affect-regulating parts of himself. He, like his adopted and deprived mother, and his son, who was adopted in fantasy, felt constantly in danger of being emotionally abandoned. Because he felt that his expectable dependence on others was tenuous, he had not developed sufficient neutralizing and regulatory ego capacities and thus felt he could not now depend on himself.

Another vicissitude of avoidant relatedness is what I would call a selective decathexis, first described to me by Susan Betts (personal communication, February 1992). Selective decathexis occurs when the parent hypercathects one part of the developing child's personality while simultaneously decathecting a reciprocal part of the child's personality. For example, some highly intelligent children become gawky and physically uncoordinated. According to Betts, the parents of such children often show great interest in their children's mental and intellectual abilities from infancy onward but treat their bodies with indifference. Betts hypothesized that such unusually bright children have, as neonates, been "held intellectually"; that is, they have not been cradled in their mother's arms but have been held upright facing the mother, as though about to have a verbal conversation. These mothers relate to the baby from the chin up and selectively deemphasize the baby's body. These children progress intellectually but selectively decathect their own bodies, which leads to physical awkwardness and spotty mind–body integration. The patient I described earlier in this chapter, who developed a learning disability after his mother paid no attention to his precocious comprehension of her infidelity and even actively encouraged his avoidance of knowledge, is another example of the effect of selective decathexis. The internalization of experiences of decathected relatedness leads to varieties of decathexis of the self. Decathexis of the self is manifested as panic about or disregard of the signals being given by one's own emotions or one's own body, and leads to varieties of affect dysregulation, psychosomatic vulnerability, and a chaotic or withdrawn relationship to one's own self.

CHAPTER ELEVEN

On the Repetition Compulsion

B ECAUSE SO MUCH OF what is deeply disturbing appears to be powerfully repetitive, a means of comprehending the repetition compulsion is especially critical for the psychoanalytic therapist. No treatment can properly be called therapeutic that does not in some fundamental way diminish the stereotypical recurrence of the individual's particular source of disquiet. Gedo (1979, 1991), however, asserted that since the general rejection of Freud's (1920) notion of a death instinct, set forward in "Beyond the Pleasure Principle," "no alternative [has] been offered that . . . [brings] the phenomena of the repetition compulsion into the realm of explanation provided by the drive theory" (1991, p. 21).

However, as I hope to describe in this chapter, recent developments in infant research may in fact offer an explanatory alternative with similar scope and better correlation with contemporary psychoanalytic practice. In particular, I suggest that the infant developmental model leads to two modifications in the way we think of the repetition compulsion: (1) The individual is compelled to repeat not only past wishes, conflicts, and traumatic experiences but the entire pattern of archaic affect regulation, which was originally mediated by the infant's mother; thus, it is not only psychopathology that is repeated but past developmental successes as well. (2) The compulsion to repeat is a prestructured interactional schema that is premotivational.

REPETITION OF THE ENTIRE PATTERN
OF ARCHAIC AFFECT REGULATION

In "Beyond the Pleasure Principle" Freud (1920) introduced the concept of the protective shield against stimuli. He defined the protective shield as the organism's "outermost surface," which "becomes to some degree inorganic and thenceforward functions as a special envelope or membrane resistant to stimuli" (p. 27).

If we extrapolate Freud's hypothesis from its economic context into a context of pre-object relatedness, the psychological protective shield can be understood to be derived from the infant's good-enough mother, who endeavors to maintain her baby's physical and emotional homeostasis. While she certainly is not inorganic, she is ultimately "non-self" and, increasingly, is subjectively perceived as such by the infant. In this sense the "outermost surface" represented by the protective shield is equivalent to a contact boundary between the skins of infant and mother. As I described in Chapter Eight, this contact boundary functions as a containing envelope or membrane, a "skin ego" (Anzieu, 1989) within which the self feels protected enough to function optimally. Bick (1968) was the first to extend Freud's metaphor of the protective shield to the prestages of object relationships:

> In its most primitive form the parts of the personality are felt to have no binding force amongst themselves and must therefore be held together in a way that is experienced by them passively, by the skin functioning as a boundary. But this internal function of containing the parts of the self is dependent initially on the introjection of an external object, experienced as capable of fulfilling this function. (p. 484)

Bick described how varieties of disturbance in the infant–mother interaction interfere with the optimal development of this containing function of the ego. Freud (1920) led the way to such a conclusion when he wrote: "We describe as 'traumatic' any excitations from outside which are powerful enough to break through the protective shield. It seems to me that the concept of trauma necessarily implies a connection of this kind with a breach in an otherwise efficacious barrier against stimuli" (p. 29).

The implication of this passage is that early trauma to the developing mental apparatus results when the signal-buffering functions of the infant–mother pair are inadequate to protect the infant from an overwhelming affect. Such experiences destroy the "background of safety" (Sandler, 1960a) maintained by the affect-regulating systems competence of the mother and infant. Later in life, trauma results when the now internalized affect-regulating ego competence is inadequate to protect the individual from overwhelming emotion. Unable to neutralize the distress adaptively through intrapsychic defense, the individual turns to others for assistance with affect containment. Freud (1920) explained why failures of the protective shield functioning of the original mother–infant pair or their subsequently internalized sequelae in the ego result in projective forms of externalization:

> [The living vesicle] is provided with a shield against stimuli from the external world. . . . [However,] towards the inside there can be no such shield. . . . [Because of this, a] particular way is adopted of dealing with any internal excitations which produce too great an increase of unpleasure: there is a tendency to treat them as though they were acting, not from the inside, but from the outside, so that it may be possible to bring the shield against stimuli into operation as a means of defense against them. This is the origin of projection, which is destined to play such a large part in the causation of pathological processes. (p. 29)

By overwhelming the capacity of the ego to maintain a background sense of safety, trauma occurring later in life can retroactively disturb pre-object functioning. For example, traumatic sexual abuse impairs the previously internalized protective shield functions of the ego. Regression to pre-object functioning leads to projective reexternalization of affect regulation, manifested by projective identification, enactment, drug abuse, promiscuity, perversion, and other means of seeking external sources of comfort and mediation.[1] Psychosomatic symptoms and mood disturbances may occur because of a regression to a somatic signal or because of projection into the body as an "external" container for overwhelming affect.[2]

---

[1]There is a reciprocal relationship between environmental failure and internalized disturbances in affect regulation. For example, disturbances in early parenting can sufficiently alter a child's behavior so as to render the child more likely to be sexually abused or exploited (Furman and Furman, 1984).

[2]One's own body in this case becomes equated with the mother's body, which is not distinguished from the self.

Winnicott (1959–1964) went further, asserting that later traumas can be indicative of breakdowns in the earliest phases of development:

> The original breakdown took place at a stage of dependence of the individual on parental or maternal ego-support. For this reason work is often done in therapeutics on a later version of the breakdown—say, a breakdown in the latency period, or even in early adolescence; this later version occurred when the patient had developed ego-autonomy and a capacity to be a person-having-an-illness. Behind such a breakdown there is always, however, a failure of defenses belonging to the individual's infancy or very early childhood. (p. 139)

If one considers repetition from the vantage point of infantile affect regulation, one is led to consider it as a form of pre-object signaling behavior. Infants tone down their overwhelming physical and emotional discomforts through amodal internalization of the soothing repetitive interactions with their caregivers. Affect regulation is accomplished in the intrapsychic sphere through these repetitive internalizations, which eventually enable the infant to send a signal of danger from one part of its developing ego to another in order to institute a defensive operation in thought. This intrapsychic defense is modeled on what was originally the systems interaction of the infant–mother pair prior to the development of the infant's capacity to mentally differentiate and symbolize whole object relations. Eugenio Gaddini (1982), referring specifically to acting out, described it as the representative of an early prerepresentational mental organization:

> As such, it is a normal phenomenon, which precedes the development of language, and of reality-oriented action and activity. Later on, it may instead establish itself as a defense. Defensive acting out seems linked to pathology in the primitive non-integrated organization of the mind, which may be able not only to prevent early ego development towards reality and object relationship, but to compel the ego to put its developing capacities in the service of the self's needs—above all, the need to survive. (p. 63)

In his paper on repression Freud (1915b) asserted that defense in its most primitive form interferes with ideational representation. Other authors have elaborated on this theory. Dorpat (1985, 1991;

Dorpat and Miller, 1992) demonstrated how psychic pain deriving from pathogenic early object relationships leads to an arrest of higher-level cognitive processes; the individual fills in the subsequent gaps in mentation with fantasies, ideas, and affects that serve a screen function. According to Kinston and Cohen (Cohen and Kinston, 1983; Kinston and Cohen, 1986), such events are related to primal repression resulting in focal failure to generate representational thought. Asserting that mental representation in the form of a wish is *created* by a need that has been met, they argued that "failure in need mediation . . . [results] in a persistent absence of associated wishes (internal self/object relations) and thus a gap in emotional understanding (psychic structure). Such a failure . . . [is] the essence of trauma" (Kinston and Cohen, 1986, p. 337).

Kinston and Cohen described how trauma deriving from failure to have needs met leads to a persistent "wound" in one's capacity for representational thought and memory about the trauma: a "hole" in one's self-experience. Is the "cognitive arrest" during denial that Dorpat referred to derived from a primary identification with the object's failure to recognize and respond to an affective need? Asking how memories are kept unconscious, Kinston and Cohen (1983) posed a radically simple answer: *There is no memory.*[3]

> The patient is in a mental state which is not structured as a memory. . . . The state observed in the analysis has been perpetuated precisely because it reflects unmet needs, that is to say, personal urges which demanded but have not obtained adequate mediation. The analyst, in dealing with the state, in effect mediates the needs and so they become represented as structured experience. Lifting of repression is therefore equivalent to repair of psychic structure. (Cohen and Kinston, 1983, p. 415)

Affects that cannot find adequate mediation leading to verbal or symbolic representation are often expressed somatically since pre-object relatedness depends on body ego functioning. As such, pathology of affect and need mediation figures prominently in the etiology of psychosomatic states, perversions (Khan 1979a, b), addictions and substance abuse, phobias, panic states, posttraumatic

---

[3]Cohen and Kinston cited Freud as the source of this idea. Freud (1940) wrote that what is meant by the term *unconscious memory* is the occurrence of something "of which we are totally unable to form a conception" (p. 197).

disorders, and self-mutilation. Gould (1991), for example, related perversion not to disorders of sexual behavior per se but to an inability to master overwhelming affects related to childhood trauma: "What distinguishes perversion is its quality of desperation and fixity. A perversion is performed by a person who has no other choices, a person who would otherwise be overwhelmed by anxieties or depression or psychosis. . . . Perversions . . . prevail over these otherwise devastating emotional states" (p. 10).

Gould (1991) argued that, viewed in these terms, perversions are suffered by females as well as males:

> A perversion is a psychological strategy. It differs from other mental strategies in that it demands a performance. The overall strategy operates in the same way for males and females. What makes all the differences between the male and female perversions is the social gender stereotype that is brought into the foreground of the enactment. The enactment, or performance, is designed to help the person to survive, moreover to survive with a sense of triumph over the traumas of his or her childhood. The perverse strategy is unconscious. The actor . . . knows only that he feels compelled to perform the perverse act and that when deterred from doing so he feels desperately anxious, panicky, agitated, crazy, even violent. The protagonist does not know that the performance is designed to master "events" that were once too exciting, too frightening, too mortifying to master in childhood. The performer cannot, dare not, remember those terrible events. Instead, his life is given up to reliving them, albeit in a disguised, symbolic form. (pp. 10–11)

The establishment of a sense of safety and hope in the psychoanalytic situation is often both deeply relieving and yet simultaneously excruciating to the patient. Frequently, after the deep experience of being understood (e.g., after the accurate interpretation of reconstructed early trauma or deprivation), the early traumatic pattern of relatedness is enacted in and out of the psychoanalytic situation. The enactment takes a variety of forms: accidents, real and psychosomatic physical illness, sleep disturbance, nightmares, panic, an exacerbation of addictive states (including substance abuse and addictive sexuality), and suicidality. Although the enactment is a signal, the connection between the patient's symptom and the activated danger state cannot be proven because the patient usually relates no symbolic links to the source of the repetition. The links, such as they exist, are presymbolic, physical, and prepsychological. They must be inferred circumstantially.

The repetition compulsion is a function of the species' progressive maturational thrust inasmuch as it provides the opportunity for past traumas to be successively worked through in subsequent developmental stages. The compulsion to repeat good-enough experiences of affect mediation by the intervention of the pre-object caregiver is the archaic substrate for the working through process in analysis. The patient's search for insight, understanding, and affect mediation in analysis is no less a compulsion to repeat past developmental successes than is psychopathology a compulsion to repeat past traumatic derailments of development.

PREMOTIVATIONAL ASPECTS
OF THE REPETITION COMPULSION

The individual does not repeat in order to master, does not enact in order to avoid thinking. These may be the *effects* of the repetition, but they should not be confused with causes. The mental apparatus that conceives unconscious wishes and other motivational structures is a moment-by-moment creation. Motivational structures are derived from the constant background repetition of archaic patterns of internal support, patterns that enable the ego to generate representational thought and meaning and to tolerate and sustain emotional pain and contact with reality. Trauma leads to the destruction of this capacity to generate thought and sustain emotion.

The interactional system of signaling another and then subsequently internalizing their adaptive emotional response is an archaic, premotivational means of regulating one's affects. The nature of the signal that is communicated is intermodal, and its reception, comprehension, and mediation by another, as well as its subsequent reinternalization in transmuted form, are often carried out intermodally. Concrete intermodal exchanges characterize pre-object relatedness. In this pre-object dimension of expression the body has its own presymbolic language of signals. The body language is presymbolic because signals are more like flags or semaphores than symbols. Because of the nature of signals, there is a concrete equivalence between one's affect and its expression in body language, whether the expression is psychosomatic (via smooth muscle) or behavioral (via striated muscle). Having developed through such pre-object forms of communication to symbolic thought and communication, adults retain an innate capacity to receive, apprehend, and transmit such interactional communications amodally. At the pre-object level of experience the repetitive behavior or psychosomatic symptom constitutes an interactional signal of impending trauma. The individual's anticipation of potential retraumatization triggers repetition of the entire pattern of archaic affect mediation.

The pre-object dimension of experience is not subsumed by later developmental processes but participates actively in them as the amodal, emotional, and psychophysiological foundation on which all representational thought is constructed. Pre-object functioning is the necessary experiential foundation for all later developmental processes. Disturbances in the pre-object level of functioning reverberate through all later developmental epochs. This suggests that an understanding of the repetition compulsion from the standpoint of pre-object functioning will apply not only to traumatic experiences of infancy but in some measure to traumatic experiences whose source is in any later developmental period. It is likely that, even though the conflict in a repetition compulsion may not itself be developmentally archaic, there may inevitably be an archaic element to the nature of the repetition itself. The archaic element is present because a psychophysiological event, for example, an affect, is the "carrier" of the subjective experience. While one's affects may be evoked by or may themselves evoke memory, fantasy, defense, and other activities based on representational thought, the underlying affect itself is a bodily sensation whose nature is more developmentally archaic than that of mental representation.

By way of explanation, let us think for a moment about the color blue (Gass, 1976). A color, as a quality of the representational world, carries symbolic meaning. We may invest thoughts of sadness (feeling blue, singing the blues) or sexual excitement (blue movie) with qualities associated with "blueness," and the color blue may make us feel sad or cold or empty or tranquil. These would be the symbolic, representable, object-related meanings of blueness. At the same time, the color blue as a visual percept is not necessarily reducible or representable by anything else. The color is a quality of lived experience that is ontologically earlier than any abstraction of blueness as a word or concept. True, we may conjure a mental picture of the color blue, and the particular shade we see in our mind's eye is a representation or memory. But the color blue itself is not an abstraction; it is concrete. In pre-object experience blue is a wavelength of the visible spectrum, not a thought. The color is meaningless before it is invested with meaning and symbolized by the representational world. Developmentally, the infant cannot invest the color blue with meaning apart from the context of an environment that mediates the attribution of meanings and so enables the infant to create thought, that is, to paint the internal world with a spectrum of colors, affects, and relationships. Yet this concrete, pre-object aspect of blue that is devoid of symbolic meaning participates in all later representational thoughts of "blue." So too with the physical sensations of affect, which, developing in the infant's awareness prior to the mental representations of affect states and prior to symbolic, verbal thought, thus have an underlying pre-object dimension.[4]

The earliest representation of an affect is amodal, concrete, and psychosomatic, not symbolic. It is premental and transmitted to others by intermodal exchange. This suggests the possibility that, even *after* the development of representational thought, individuals need not intend, consciously or unconsciously, for their behavior to be a signal to another. The newborn need not be capable of mentally representing its distress in order to communicate its overwhelmed state to its mother. According to Max Stern (1988):

> We must conceive trauma as the result of a lack of information necessary to the accomplishment of a developmentally functional performance. If the performance is the maintenance of homeostatic equilibrium in the very young infant, then the missing information can be conceptualized . . . as the lack of the holding and soothing presence of the mother who vouchsafes that equilibrium. (p. 144)

Stern challenged Freud's assertion that a wish for mastery is revealed in the repetition of traumatic experiences. He claimed that, when mastery cannot be provided by the human surround or generated by the developmentally arrested personality, "the traumatic

---

[4]Ogden (1989a, b) has given a particularly moving personal description of the emotional panic that ensues in a regression to the pre-object state, where symbolic meanings lose their linkage to words, which then become concrete, meaningless sounds.

event is repeated not in order to be mastered, but *because it is the nature of the performance to remember"* (p. 144; emphasis added).

Describing the signal function of the repetition, Stern also conceptualized, as I do, signal affects in the broader context of human relatedness when he asserted that "the function of that defense [of the nervous system against shock] remains paramount . . . in providing a signal, in the form of agitated behavior to the human surround and in the form of primary depression to the individual, of the need for external assistance in the face of disorganizing states of tension" (p. 147). For example, Stern's description of traumatic dreams is as follows:

> In the absence of preparedness for danger, the subject will revert—indeed, regress—to the method of working employed by the mental apparatus in its earliest efforts at mastery. His dreams will thus persist until adaptation to the consequences of the trauma has occurred—that is, until signal anxiety can be brought to bear on the memory of the traumatic situation. (pp. 112–113)

Stern claimed, citing the geneticist Monod, that for the human species the inevitable experience of trauma is necessary for the development of the capacity for anticipation. For example, he saw pavor nocturnus as a compulsion to repeat in the service of overcoming a developmental failure to attribute meaning to states of tension. In light of the views advanced here, I would add that such an experience does not so much derive from the failure to attribute meaning as from the functional *inability* to attribute meaning. This is an important distinction theoretically since one of the criticisms of the concept of projective identification is that it supposes a motivational and representational capacity in infants that is generally thought to develop only later. Ogden (1979) attempted to remove this objection by modifying the theory so as to move the onset of the capacity for projective identification forward developmentally. While this strategy solves one theoretical problem, it dilutes the powerful explanatory value of the concept of projective identification as the prototype for the earliest form of human affect regulation. The concept of intermodal exchange addresses this theoretical problem by presenting the possibility of direct sensorimotor transfer of affect-modifying ego functions without the intermediary of ideational thought. Intermodal exchange is the developmental substrate of the differentiated representational transformations necessary for projective identification proper. Intermodal exchanges can be triggered directly, without the intervening motivated unconscious wish or fantasy of externalizing one's overwhelming affects into another person or into an internal object representation.

This model of archaic affect regulation based on intermodal exchange is supported by the recognition that supramodal representational capacities exist at or shortly after birth, capacities that enable the caregiver to assist the neonate in regulating its traumatically overwhelming affect states. It is not necessary to assume that neonates must have already developed the motivational capacity to wish to induce in their caregivers adaptive responses to their trauma in order for their behavioral repetition to have this effect.

CHAPTER TWELVE

Trauma and Enactment

ANYTHING DESERVING THE NAME trauma is emotionally overwhelming and is thus experienced as indistinguishable from states of disorganization in infancy in which adequate mediation by the environment was absent. Trauma duplicates states of experience prior to which the personality could not generate meaning, because the attribution of meaning relies on a symbolic capacity that traumatic ego disorganization obliterates. In the pre-object state, meaning is attributed by the auxiliary ego functioning of the caregiver who receives and mediates the individual's distress signal, not by the individual whose emotional distress acts as the signal. In the pre-object dimension of communication, affect and meaning are evoked in another intermodally via interactional enactment rather than conveyed symbolically in verbal speech.

Because of this, there will be times when the therapist, as mediator of the patient's affects in the transference, is compelled to repeat the patient's past no less than the patient. There are two corollaries to this view. The first corollary is that where there is a paucity of actual experience of developmental success, there will be a disturbed capacity for the working alliance to sustain and ameliorate the traumatic enactments that the treatment will revive. The second corollary is that the patient is, in some measure, also compelled to repeat the traumas and successes of the *therapist's* past. The therapeutic situation is structured to tilt the balance of repetition in the direction of the patient's inner world and to maximize the opportunities for understanding the nature of that inner world, but the ultimate nature of the enactment is in some ways a compromise formation between the internal worlds of the two participants.

While this mutual enactment may lead to pathology of the therapeutic situation, it also underlies one of the central therapeutic aspects of the treatment situation: The patient, in a small way, reenacts the developmental successes of the analyst and gradually internalizes the therapist's more mature and adaptive response to the patient's enacted traumas.

In a panic, a psychotic patient phoned me as well as his relatives one Sunday afternoon, seemingly desperate to reestablish contact. He had begun to hallucinate angry accusatory voices that called him all kinds of repellent names. At the next session we were able to trace the source of his panic, with resulting considerable relief for the patient. What we learned was that the previous week he had made a rare attempt to assert himself with his mother and, as a result, felt that his mother had threatened to terminate their relationship. This was related in the treatment situation to my having previously canceled his Monday appointment. That Sunday, the day he usually visited with his mother and the day before the canceled appointment, he had been in a panic all day. Until the session he was unable to be aware of the source of his panic in his inability to be with his mother or me. His rage made him frightened for our safety and for the safety of his attachments to us, although he experienced this fear primarily as a terror that he was falling to pieces.

When talking about his panic during the next session he described the nature of the voices he had started to hear the day before. I said that hearing the upsetting voices outside of him indicated that he was not aware of what was upsetting inside of him. He said, "That's why I smoke so much when I'm upset."

I immediately felt an intuitive sense of having understood perfectly what he meant, and he gave me an odd little smile. A second later I realized that his statement made no obvious logical sense. I said that I did not quite understand the connection he was drawing between smoking and hallucination. He smiled again at me and said, "Well, *you* know . . . " and then, by way of example, he blew loudly from his mouth as if exhaling in relief after having taken a deep drag from a cigarette and holding his breath. I realized that he was right; I *had* known. My patient was describing a forceful projective identification first described by Bion (1957). A harmful introject is split into innumerable minute particles and then forcefully extruded. The particles then lead a quasi-independent existence as a hallucinatory voice, as with this man, or as a hovering cloud of smoke.

Although I had initially understood the patient, this capacity to understand him had made me anxious about the archaic elements in my own personality. I had then fled from this primitive understanding to more rational thought processes.

The patient's hallucinations on that painful Sunday could be traced to the traumatic effect on his ego functioning of his experience of his mother's avoidance of the vital form of contact and affect regulation he required and to my similar avoidance in the ensuing transference–countertransference enactment. In the patient's metaphor, exhaling could be construed as a wish to project noxious internal contents into the surround and perhaps even as a sadistic wish to thereby foul the air for others. However, the man's subsequent comment, "Well, *you* know . . . " seems to substantiate the notion that the projective aspects of pre-object forms of affect regulation are premotivational. It would be physiologically impossible *not* to exhale, whether one wanted to or not. Developmentally, the fantasies that accompany projective identification might represent first attempts to think about and to embody within the realm of one's omnipotence the involuntary externalizing actions of pre-object affect regulation.

In the view presented here the repetition compulsion, as it becomes manifest in the therapeutic situation, is the inevitable result of a regression of affect regulation from internalized methods to externalized ones that are characteristic of pre-object relatedness. The intermodal exchanges of pre-object relatedness predate wishes, which require symbolic mental representations. Through behavioral repetition triggered by the transference relationship the individual utilizes intermodal exchanges that temporarily bolster those ego capacities whose functioning has been destabilized. However, the pre-object substrate of this activity may involve no more motivation or wishfulness than does the reflex of a knee hit by a physician's mallet. Did this man want or intend to hallucinate when he felt his mother and I were foreclosing a vital means of affect regulation to him? Does a knee want or intend to master the effect of the doctor's blow by jerking?

COUNTERTRANSFERENCE AS REPETITION

Through the repetition compulsion an individual signals to others the existence of inner disturbances that cannot be adequately neutralized, or even contemplated, by purely intrapsychic means. As such, the repetition compulsion can be conceived of as a form of momentary regression to externalized forms of affect regulation that are characteristic of pre-object relatedness. In the adult such externalization takes the form of behavioral enactment triggered by similar affect-saturated experiences later in life. It is these affects, embedded in pre-object contexts of relatedness (Emde, 1988a) prior to the development of autonomous affect regulation, that serve as the original signal of danger to which Freud referred. Derived from primary relatedness, the signal of danger is not internalized or symbolized; nor is it under ego control. It is a signal that can only be expressed in action and can only be understood by a caregiver. Enactment demands mediation from the environment in order to create a semblance of an internal world that can encompass the affect. Without such environmental mediation there is no inner support for the moment-by-moment creation of mental representations, internalized object relationships, ego defenses, drive neutralization, and reality testing.

In the context of pre-object relations, behavioral repetition can be understood as a signal function of the ego that indicates a regression in the individual's affect-regulating capacities. When an individual's intrapsychic defenses are temporarily overwhelmed, there is a depletion of the resources and stimulus barrier functions of protective objects and the parts of one's ego that have internalized their regulatory functions. The individual must desperately search for an individual in the environment who can adequately receive the communicated danger signal and supplement the neutralizing capacity of his or her ego. In analysis or psychoanalytic therapy this individual is the therapist, the transference is the medium of enacted communication, and the therapist's therapeutic technique and handling of countertransference are the carriers of the requisite mediation. Cohen and Kinston (1983) stated unequivocally that "the analyst is therefore called upon to mediate as well as interpret during the process of working through. Mediation is required to enable representation of needs and growth of psychic structures. This mediation is not a parameter but an inherent part of the analytic relationship" (p. 419).

The patient is compelled to seek out this mediation of traumatic states in the analysis, to experience a background of safety as though for the first time in relation to his overwhelming distress:

The patient was a man who manifested an intense a form of withdrawn relatedness. Needless to say, the man's ambivalence about closeness and distance had been enacted and explored many times before in the analysis. The Wednesday session had been characteristic of a recent sea change that seemed to be occurring in the analysis: The patient was gradually becoming more emotionally alive, that is, warmer and more emotionally available. When I ended the session he got up and said on his way out the door, "See you . . . ," and his voice trailed off, leaving him looking confused. I imagined that he was not certain what day of the week it was and therefore whether he would see me the next day or Monday. He finally recalled that it was Wednesday, looked relieved, added the word "tomorrow" to his sentence, and left.

The next day the patient began by saying, "I had a hard time leaving the office yesterday." What he meant was that he had *literally* had a hard time after leaving because he had gotten stuck in a traffic jam. Moreover, there had been a state trooper in the car behind him, and despite numerous single-occupant cars whizzing by in the car pool lane the police officer did nothing to stop them, which had irritated my patient. He then spoke about his plans to be alone over the upcoming weekend rather than spending it with his woman friend. As the session proceeded, he became increasingly withdrawn, morose, alienated, and concrete. I realized that my mind had begun to wander in a kind of counterwithdrawal. I took my withdrawal as a cue and spoke.

I drew the patient's attention back to his opening statement and asked if there had been other reasons, besides the traffic jam, for the difficulty he had had leaving the office on the previous day. I mentioned that he had appeared confused as he left, as though he had not been certain whether we were scheduled to meet the next day or not. He said, "Yes, I was confused about that. But I was also confused about something else. I was wearing a heavy overshirt. When I got up to leave, I looked on the chair for it and discovered it wasn't there. Then I looked on the coat hook for it, and it wasn't there either. Finally, I realized that I was wearing it already. I was so perplexed about that that I forgot what day it was." In this way, the search for a mediating object that might have been lost or might have been (almost) internalized made it possible for the man to begin to talk about his fear of missing me and his girlfriend over the upcoming weekend break.

I asked if yesterday's appointment had created a hard time for him in other ways as well. Had he felt, for example, that I, who, like the trooper, was behind him, was also in some way negligent? After some thought he replied, "I thought I heard you making some noise during the session. I wondered if you were paying attention and listening to me."

"So you *were* like the trooper," he continued. "Not just because you sit behind me but also because I noticed in the rearview mirror that the trooper was looking away distractedly. He wasn't paying attention, so he didn't notice what was going on. He couldn't respond to the situation." The patient's mood had begun to improve, and he was no longer thinking concretely.

I wondered if the lost shirt related to what he felt was his original loss of the protective shield functions of his mother in the first few months of life. He was reexperiencing this loss in the analysis. This protective shield was gradually being repaired when he sensed I was adequately related to him. It was damaged again when he sensed that I was not paying attention. This crucial early loss of adequate affect mediation was recreated and repeated in the analytic interaction through intermodal exchange; it was the primal trauma he was compelled to repeat endlessly. The patient referred obliquely to this early experience when he suffered a momentary disturbance of ego functioning (affecting cognition and memory) at the end of the previous session and when he concretely confused the analyst with the protective functioning of his overshirt.

The cooling system of an automobile provides an apt metaphor for these processes, albeit one that is, unfortunately, mechanistic. As long as the temperature of the coolant in the system remains within the capacities of the system, the entire volume of the coolant remains within the confines of the system (internalized, as it were). However, as the temperature of the coolant rises its volume expands until the system can no longer contain it in its entirety. In older automobiles, this resulted in pressure building up within the system. Sometimes the coolant would boil over and be lost. As coolant was progressively lost, the cooling capacity of the system was diminished, necessitating occasional replacement of coolant. More modern automobiles have a sealed cooling system that prevents boiling over. In this more advanced system the internal cooling system is dynamically connected to a small overflow tank. When the temperature of the coolant rises, pressure does not build up because the expanding coolant can spill over, out of the internalized container into the external container. As the system cools progressively, the coolant's volume contracts and the external container empties back into the cooling system.

The vintage automobile cooling system is analogous to pre-object affect regulation. Physical and emotional upsets overwhelm the individual's capacity to think and so to mediate his or her own emotional discomforts, resulting in behavioral enactment and storms of incapacitating affect that cannot adequately be represented. Adequate environmental provision, adapted to the patient's needs through the mediation of the therapist, maximizes the patient's efforts to regulate his own affects. Patients repeatedly make use of their analyst's therapeutic assistance and later, after internalizing this ability to assist their own ego functioning, become gradually better able to represent the trauma as object-related thought and thus to control and regulate their own biological processes and affects.

The ways of containing and regulating intrapsychic conflict are as follows:

1. *Internal defense*: At the most mature level, one manages the fluctuations of one's own conflicts and emotions in terms of internalized ego defenses and the modulated regulation of one's own emotions. Such conflict is quite amenable to being thought of in terms of Freud's structural theory. The conflict is experienced intrapsychically in relation to repressed unconscious wishes and occurs between intact psychic structures and whole, differentiated internal objects.

2. *Fantasy of externalization*: When this effort is insufficient, one utilizes the fantasy of projection into internal objects. One fantasies the containing, neutralizing, supporting, and stimulus barrier functions these internalized objects provide and fantasies being freed (via projection) from the

conflictual feelings and wishes. Defenses involving fantasies of externalization are characteristic of, but not limited to, the latency phase of development (Etchegoyen, 1993).

3. *Transitional*: The emotional pain is extruded through the use of transitional objects. However, since transitional objects are not clearly differentiated for the self, the boundaries between externalization and internalization may be blurred. For example, some people will buy themselves something to ward off a mild depressive affect or will play the radio in their automobiles to avert an unconscious feeling of loneliness (Winnicott, 1958b).

4. If these measures fail, one's recourse is to ambivalent or avoidant relatedness:

   a. *Ambivalent relatedness*: Ambivalent relatedness is characterized by the failure of the ego to adequately receive signal anxiety, a failure that leads to panic states and pathological projective identification. The individual desperately "evacuates" or "dumps" the affect onto or into an external object through intermodal exchange, sometimes eliciting an adaptive response.

   b. *Avoidant relatedness*: Pervasive depression, schizoid states, or alexithymia fail to develop further that aspect of the ego that could experience the overwhelming affect and progressively deplete the compensatory supply lines of pleasure as described by Weil (1992).

At first glance it seems that at more neurotic levels of development the individual is able to process the emotional disturbance intrapsychically, while at more borderline or psychotic levels of development the individual processes the disturbance interactionally. This view grows out of the prevalent notion that the hallmark of higher-level defenses (such as repression, reaction formation, and undoing) is that they operate between intact intrapsychic structures whereas the hallmark of lower-level or "primitive" defenses (such as splitting, denial, and projective identification) is that they are interactional and operate between self and object in external reality. In actuality, however, this distinction is often absent. First of all, the affect regression (Krystal, 1988) inherent in defense against anticipated trauma may itself be sufficient to shift the register of experience toward a pre-object mode, at least momentarily. In addition, as Freud (1926) first demonstrated in "Inhibitions, Symptoms and Anxiety," even the most differentiated levels of ego functioning rely on signaling activity inasmuch as one part of the ego is signaling another part of the ego for a mediating response. Finally, even though mature affect regulation is ostensibly taking place internally via ego defense, not even the most mature individual—not even the person who has achieved the most secure state of self- and object constancy—can function long or well without the ongoing interactional and emotional support of significant others. Therefore, the more psychotherapeutically relevant question may be not what the DSM diagnosis of the individual is but at what developmental level of cognition and affect regulation the individual is functioning *at that moment*. Diagnoses tend to describe the probability of functional level. For example, it is obvious that neurotics generally tend to function at a higher level than do psychotics. However, at any given moment the so-called psychotic individual may be functioning at a highly integrated and lucid level while the so-called neurotic may be in a state of momentary regression to highly primitive experience. Functional level is a dynamic aspect of personality functioning and can therefore be affected moment by moment by the interplay of internal reality with the experience of the adequacy of environmental support and mediation.

To cite just one developmental example of the relativity of functional level, Mahler, Pine, and Bergman (1975), describing the spurt in autonomous functioning that begins with the development of upright locomotion, called the time between the ages of 10 and 18 months a "love affair with the world." The child's abilities shift rapidly in the direction of his or her newfound autonomy. The child avidly explores his or her body and other objects in an expanding environment, manifests a relative imperviousness to frustrations and bumps, and accepts substitute adults easily. Yet the child's capacity to maintain this excited drive toward autonomy lasts only as long as the adequacy of parental attunement can be taken for granted. If the mother is not optimally available, the independence of the toddler soon collapses into tears and frustrated rage. The child's "autonomy" is not autonomous but is a partial internalization of a pre-object relationship with the good-enough mother.

Briefly consulting me early in my career was a man who

manifested this regression of affect regulation to externalized means, which is inherent in the repetition compulsion:

> I was once asked by a company to perform a psychiatric evaluation of Mr. A, a man having work-related problems. The day prior to the appointment Mr. A knocked on the exterior door of my office, interrupting an appointment. When I opened the door, Mr. A quickly introduced himself as the man I'd be meeting the next day and handed me a large, heavy box. He said, "If you want to understand my situation you'll have to read all of this before you talk with me tomorrow." Mr. A added, almost as an afterthought, "Please be careful with these papers. I didn't have the time to copy them because I only received the notice of the appointment from the company today. These are my only copies." Then he turned and left.
>
> Because of the urgency of the intrusion, I opened his package that evening with some curiosity. There were 400–500 pages of original typewritten material, copies of newspaper reports, and court transcripts. The information included past medical evaluations, transcripts of hearings, and research studies concerning the emotional stresses faced by other employees whose particular work responsibilities coincided with those of Mr. A. Pertinent excerpts were meticulously underlined, apparently in order to make the task of reading more manageable for me. I began to read, planning to give the material only a cursory review.
>
> The court depositions made clear that Mr. A had an exemplary work history until he took a position with identical responsibilities in a new company. At the new job he began to notice severe safety defects, which he reported. Not only were the defects not corrected, but he was reprimanded for making the complaints. Over a period of several years, an escalating spiral developed in which Mr. A increasingly assumed the role of whistle-blower. He repeatedly reported potentially life-threatening safety deficiencies, and his alarms were generally ignored. He was seen as a troublemaker, and he was eventually demoted despite good performance appraisals. He felt overwhelmed by the constant fear of a deadly accident. He began to develop severe anxiety, social withdrawal, sleeplessness, loss of memory, rashes, an exaggerated startle response, a fear of reprisals by his supervisors, and an intense preoccupation with

thoughts relating to work. The psychiatrists who had previously examined him for the company had all concluded that he was a paranoid individual engaged in a vendetta against the company. He then initiated grievance proceedings, which dragged on through years of review, culminating in my appointment with him the next day. By the time I put his records away and closed the lid of the box, I realized that I had spent the entire evening reading, instead of the ten minutes I had planned.

The man was punctual for the interview the following day. He was quite guarded and withdrawn, speaking cautiously and primarily in answer to direct questions. On more than one occasion he looked startled and very nearly jumped when I asked him an unexpected question. He said, "I was a dedicated individual, good at my job, and concerned about safety. There were situations there that were potentially life threatening. I feel the company has been unfair; they've lost whole files of mine. I feel like I'm attached to it, like I can't get away from it. I feel like I can't move. I feel inhibited and restrained. I'm having to lead an altered life, I have this thing that rides around on my shoulder all the time. All I want to do is to set the record straight."

As he was talking I suddenly believed I understood why he had interrupted me the day before: I had felt that it was impossible for me to read and assimilate 400 pages in only one evening and he had felt that it was impossible for him to assimilate the life and death responsibilities of his job. His actions had unconsciously given me an inkling of the same sort of overwhelming burden in my responsibilities concerning him that he had felt in his job. In a small way he was intruding upon and overwhelming me just as he had felt intruded upon and overwhelmed.

Accordingly, I said to him, "I think you have been feeling overwhelmed by these events. You can't distance yourself from them or let go of them, and you have perhaps been hoping that I could have some inkling of what it must feel like to you." To my surprise, the man immediately burst into tears and sobbed uncontrollably. He wept for the remaining time of the appointment, overwhelmed by his emotions. He was moving to another city shortly, but continued to maintain occasional contact with me for years afterward.

Now, clearly, the remarkable sense of detachment this man exhibited belied an overwhelming sense of panic and despair, which he could not ordinarily express in verbal or symbolic terms. He was detached because he could not find an object in external reality or any part of his self in internal reality who could receive his projected feeling of being overwhelmed and persecuted. My initial lack of understanding repeated his trauma. When I eventually managed to find the balanced response he needed, a response that indicated to him that I could tolerate and understand his suffering, that I was open to his intermodal exchange of emotion, he was able to create within his own mind a capacity to think about and to express his overwhelming affects.

At these times, then, the therapist will reenact in advance of understanding. In fact, one means of understanding archaic states is by paying attention to the nature and sensations of one's reenactments. In this way the developmental basis of the negative transference can be thought of as the compulsion for patient and therapist to repeat the failures of earliest development, and the developmental basis of the working alliance can be thought of as their compulsion to repeat the successes of the self-regulating others who could mediate those traumas and enable them to be endured.

CHAPTER THIRTEEN

Incorrect Interpretation and the Reconstruction of Infantile Trauma

Affective states have become incorporated in the
mind as precipitates of primaeval traumatic
experiences, and when a similar situation occurs
they are revived like mnemic symbols.
—*Sigmund Freud,*
"Inhibitions, Symptoms and Anxiety"

In this work the failures of the therapist . . . will be
real and they can be shown to reproduce the
original failures, in token form.
—*D. W. Winnicott,*
"Psychotherapy of Character Disorders"

PSYCHOANALYTIC INTERPRETATIONS arise out of uncertainty. An analyst cannot know precisely in advance either the accuracy or the effect of his or her interpretations, because interpretations are conjectures about the unconscious. Only the patient's response to the interpretation confirms or fails to confirm it. Despite the analyst's lengthy training, years of clinical experience, and good intentions, his interpretations may be incorrect.

Because of the importance of correct and timely interpretation to the therapeutic action of psychoanalysis, the literature concerning it is justifiably large and seemingly in constant revision. The literature concerning *in*correct interpretations is minuscule in comparison, perhaps because of the once prevalent assumption that

---

Presented July 27, 1987, at the 35th International Psychoanalytical Congress, Montreal, Canada.

incorrect interpretations do not matter very much. This opinion was already common when Edward Glover wrote his classic 1931 paper "The Therapeutic Effect of Inexact Interpretation: A Contribution to the Theory of Suggestion," in which he wrote, "A glaringly inaccurate interpretation is probably without effect unless backed by strong transference authority, but a slightly inexact interpretation may increase our difficulties." The view that incorrect interpretations are inconsequential has begun to yield only relatively recently. The change is seen in studies on the importance of the psychoanalytic setting (Loewald, 1960; Winnicott, 1958a, b, 1965, 1971a), the analyst's empathic understanding of the patient (Kohut, 1971, 1977; Schwaber, 1981; Stolorow et al., 1987), the therapist's contributions to the psychopathology of the psychoanalytic situation (Langs, 1978, 1979, 1980; Raney, 1984; Searles, 1975), and such interactional elements of psychoanalysis as projective identification (Furman, 1987; Ogden, 1979, 1982) and role responsiveness (Sandler, 1976).

Strachey (1934), in his paper on the therapeutic action of psychoanalysis, set forward a paradigm of the correct interpretation, which he described as the "mutative" interpretation. It is the nature of correct interpretations to occur on a small scale and to be directed at the "point of urgency" that exists in any given session. They are expressed by the analyst in a highly specific, detailed, and concrete manner. Because mutative interpretations primarily concern transferential aspects of the patient's relation to the analyst within a given session, they are experienced by the patient as emotionally immediate.

Strachey emphasized the need for specificity in the expression of interpretations and asserted that vagueness in interpretation bolsters the patient's resistances. To support this claim, Strachey cited Glover's paper, which had been published three years earlier. He agreed with Glover's view that only slightly inexact interpretations were pernicious and antianalytic because they enabled patients to strengthen their repression.

However, the hypothesis that an incorrect interpretation primarily strengthens the patient's repression raises a crucial question. Why would there be a strengthening of repression if the analyst's intervention, owing to its vagueness or inaccuracy, fails to release a latent instinctual component? According to drive–defense theory, any increase in the patient's use of ego defenses must be motivated by the signal function of a perceived danger situation.

The near miss of the analyst's inexact interpretation could be argued to be more likely to mitigate anxiety than to arouse it.

I believe that the answer lies in presuming that it is the incorrect interpretation itself that represents a danger to the patient. Each incorrect interpretation—and, in a larger sense, incorrect intervention of any type, whether interpretive or not, spoken or not—is experienced by the patient as a painful or frightening disillusionment that repeats, on a small scale, similar misunderstandings or failures of need mediation suffered in past relationships. Patients' reactions not only mimic their past affective responses but also recapitulate whatever defensive solutions they found to the past environmental lapse. Thus, the archaic trauma that resulted in either fixed constellations of impulse and defense, pathological character structure, cumulative trauma (Khan, 1963), developmental strain, or developmental arrest (Sandler, 1967) are reproduced in the patient's regressive response to the analyst's incorrect interpretation (and sometimes heightened) and can be reconstructed from this response.

Since the emphasis in this chapter is upon the patient's experience of interpretive errors, I choose the word *incorrect* rather than *inexact* or *incomplete* (which appear more frequently in the psychoanalytic literature) to describe such interpretations. The usual terms are primarily geared to the analyst's technical evaluation of his or her own precision, while *incorrect* refers primarily to the patient's immediate experience of the interpretation's validity. From the point of view of the regressed patient in analysis the erroneous interpretation feels wrong, if not actually false, disappointing, or hurtful. To the patient, the incorrect interpretation feels like the return of the repressed, projected into the analytic situation. Well-integrated patients feel as though the analyst has dropped the ball; poorly integrated ones feel as though they themselves have been dropped.

No criticism is intended in the recognition that psychoanalysts sometimes err in their interpretations. To be sure, many (though certainly not all) interpretive errors are initially induced through the analyst's role responsiveness to the patient's subtle pressures within the transference. Nevertheless, patients, either consciously or unconsciously, recognize their analyst's errors for what they are and react to them.

This is not to say that the patient is always consciously aware that an interpretation has been erroneous. Since such traumatic reactions reenact sometimes quite early experiences of failed emotional support for emerging ego capacities, the only manifest result of the incorrect interpretation may be a worsening of the patient's mood, a collapse of self-experience, a deterioration in the patient's condition, a weakening in the working alliance, or an explosion of enactment within the analytic hours or between sessions.[1] The unfortunate corollary of Loewald's (1960) discovery that the patient reaches a higher level of ego integration through the effect of analytic understanding is that incorrect interpretations may have a *dis*integrating effect on the patient. These momentary lapses and the ways in which the patient responds to them become part of the data of the analysis, woven into the pattern of the evolving analytic interaction. Given that analysts are human, incorrect interpretations are inevitable. But especially because of their inevitability and because they are experienced in the transference as repetitions, incorrect interpretations must be analyzed.

Such clinical deterioration should not be confused with negative therapeutic reaction (Freud, 1918, 1923, 1933). Many instances of clinical deterioration erroneously characterized as negative therapeutic reactions are actually iatrogenic sequelae of incorrect interpretations. The term "negative therapeutic reaction," then, should be reserved for a consistently untoward response to an interpretation the patient feels is genuinely correct, timely, and empathic. For example, some patients respond poorly to interventions that temporarily enable them to make a developmental advance, because in the past they experienced parental rejection or abandonment after their attempts to separate or individuate. The belief that movement toward independence was intolerably hurtful to the parent is one source of the unconscious sense of guilt Freud first postulated as generating the negative therapeutic reaction. The expected improvement reoccurs after exploration of the patient's fears that newfound gains will threaten his or her attachment to the analyst.

---

[1]One example of this type of incorrect interpretation is given by Kohut and Wolf (1978), who wrote, concerning their treatment of narcissistic patients, "Subsequent to an erroneous interpretation, however—e.g., following a session in which the analyst had addressed himself to some detail of the patient's psychic life when, in fact (after some progress in treatment, for example, or after some external success), the patient had offered his total self for approval—the patient's feeling of wholeness which had been maintained via the transference disappears" (p. 419).

EFFECTS ON THE PATIENT'S EXPERIENCE
OF SELF AND OBJECT

Basch (1985) described a developmental line of response to the analyst's interpretations. In my view, this developmental line relates to the severity, nature and timing of the developmental trauma that is reproduced by the incorrect interpretation.

The patient, a middle-aged housewife and mother in the first months of her analysis, described a recent visit by her younger sister, who was a highly successful and affluent attorney. She had arrived at the patient's home wearing designer clothing and driving a fast and expensive new sports car.

The analyst said after a while that he thought the patient was envious of her sister's wealth and success. The patient agreed, saying that she even expected the analyst might say something of that sort, given that a psychotherapist in the past had once made an interpretation to her about her bitter envy of others. She went on in a desultory manner to say that although her sister's taste in clothing was not her own, she too would like the freedom to buy anything she wanted, including expensive clothing and automobiles. While she and her husband made a comfortable living from his work and her part-time job, it was nowhere near what her sister made. The patient blamed herself for this situation: If she had concentrated on advanced schooling and had more ambitiously pursued a full-time career rather than "lazily" settling for marriage and motherhood, she too could have enjoyed a measure of her sister's affluence. She also felt dejected and ashamed to discover that she was still a mean-spirited person who could not be happy for her sister's success. She went on in this vein for a while, with darkening mood.

The analyst finally said that it sounded as if his earlier comment about her envy had resulted in her becoming quite self-critical, and he reminded her that she was accusing herself of being lazy, mean-spirited, on so on. The patient seemed quite surprised by this observation. She wondered why she had reacted with such self-criticism when, in fact, the analyst's comment about her envy had not come as much of a shock. Her envy was something she was already aware of. She eventually concluded that she had thought that the analyst's choosing to point out to her what she assumed was obvious indicated to her that perhaps *he* was critical of her for her envy. Her self-criticism followed.

The analyst said that he wondered if she had felt that his comment about her envy was not only beside the point but also somehow incorrect. The patient now responded with an immediate lifting of her previous depressive gloom and a return to her usual way of speaking. In fact, she now said, what had plagued her throughout her sister's visit was her guilt about what she felt was her sister's envy of *her* success. Her sister, the patient now said, had made many envious comments during the visit about the patient's new home, her secure family life, and her overall contentment. The patient felt somehow guilty, as if her good judgment and luck had somehow contributed to her sister's lifelong dissatisfaction. She began to remember that despite her sister's recent material success she (the patient) had always considered herself the luckier and happier of the two. Her sister had had a troubled childhood, including school problems and constant difficulties with her parents and teachers. The patient described her conflicts concerning her competitiveness with her sister dating from their childhood. Guiltily, she had always felt that she would not change places with her sister for a minute.

She had defended against this feeling by inhibiting her ordinary assertiveness and by excessive self-blame. The patient's response in the transference had been initiated and accentuated by her perception of the analyst's incorrect interpretation. While patients in therapy sometimes accuse their therapist of all manner of egregious mistakes, these conscious accusations frequently serve the purpose of resistance. In contrast, the recognition that an interpretation has been truly incorrect is frequently *denied* by the patient. The patient, identifying with the aggressor, defensively identifies with the analyst and complies with the incorrect interpretation, often at his or her own expense.

The process illustrated by this case example can be described as a defensive reversal of representational perspective, in which the patient altered her self-representation to conform to the view of her she felt was expressed by the analyst. In Chapter Six I described how even after the development of object constancy the mental images of both self and object are composite unities that can shift perspective between self and object poles. Reversal of representational perspective may occur in normal development (as in the internalization of parental values as part of the child's own self-representation), as well as defensively and psychopathologically.

This is unlike reaction formation or turning into the opposite, in which drive representations reverse polarity (e.g., love for hate) while the representations of self and object are undisturbed. In reversal of representational perspective the patient substitutes a reciprocal self-representation for the disavowed object representation, or vice versa. Patients may reverse the representational perspective between themselves and their analyst in order to disavow the pain, anxiety, and danger that recognition of the analyst's error brings and in order to preserve the link to the analyst. However, the affect representation remains the same: For example, the patient's feeling attacked or criticized by the analyst becomes transformed into self-reproach or a depressive mood. Not infrequently, what a patient primarily remembers after analysis are the incorrect interpretations, which have been defensively idealized as being true. Patients frequently rationalize their distressed reaction to the interpretation as being for their own ultimate good. In contrast, the analyst's correct interpretations, which resulted in whatever benefit the patient derived from the treatment, are largely forgotten in time. The patient feels generally grateful for the analyst's good work, but long afterward the specifics of good-enough analyzing, like the details of good-enough mothering (Winnicott, 1960a) are taken for granted and fade into the "background of safety" (Sandler, 1960a; Sandler and Sandler, 1978) of the analysis. They are forgotten because they have been internalized. In contrast, unanalyzed incorrect interpretations cannot as easily be forgotten. They may remain as introjects (Calef and Weinshel, 1981), like mental and emotional foreign bodies.

Such a reaction in some ways focally impairs patients' capacity for reality testing (Dorpat, 1985) since they are blinded to the existence of the shortcoming in the analyst insofar as the perceived shortcoming now exists within their own self-representation. Not only the scotomatized reality but also the reparative fantasy and its associated affect state must be analyzed in order to resolve the antianalytic effect of the error, since such patients have denied the actual occurrence of the analyst's error, have displaced the fault to themselves, and have identified with how they believe the analyst thinks of them. Hence, the reaction to an incorrect interpretation is related to the displacement of aggression onto the self-representation, which is in itself a reaction to the signal threat of narcissistic vulnerability. *Viewed in this light, the strengthening of the patient's defenses noted by Strachey and Glover is a secondary adaptive maneuver whose aim is to protect the self from what it feels to be a traumatic impingement by the analyst.*

THE INTERPRETATION AS TRANSITIONAL OBJECT

The patient relates to the analyst as both a transference object and a real object. Green (1978) asserted that "the aim and object of psychoanalysis is, in short, the construction of the *analytic object*, which the analysand can carry away with him from the analysis and can make use of in the absence of the analyst, who is no longer the object of transference" (p. 173; emphasis in original).

However, it seems to me that the patient relates not only to the analyst but also to the analyst's interpretations, although the interpretation is not entirely an object to the patient, as is the analyst. The patient's link to the analyst's interpretation is more developmentally primitive and relates to responses to phase-adequate holding, mirroring, and "affect attunement" (Stern, 1985 a, b). According to Bion (1967a), the analyst is ideally like an empty container for the patient's wishes, defenses, and needs. Patients induce in their analyst's empathic reverie a mirror of their own emotional and mental state, which the analyst can employ to formulate the correct interpretation. Put more simply, the patient makes the analyst aware of what the analyst needs to know in order for the analyst to be able to make the patient aware of what he or she needs to know.

Interventions may have two different effects on the patient. Some interventions act to release unconscious thoughts and affects from defensive sequestration. This type of intervention is followed by some form of externalization, either in fantasy or in action, which allows for the possibility of *external mediation* of the unconscious disturbance. In this sense, acting out can be understood as a sign of hope (Winnicott, 1963b). Some other forms of intervention prompt and assist the *internal mediation* of the unconscious contents and affects. Both forms of intervention lead eventually to the conscious emotional registering of the affect and tolerable thought about the conflict.

In a past paper (Kumin, 1989) I described how interpretations are not wholly products of the analyst but are in some sense a shared creation of the analyst and the patient. Thus, in the creation of the "analytic object" the analyst's good-enough interpretations occupy a transitional space for patients, neither fully inside nor fully outside them. This transitional object occurs in the overlap between patients' creation of the correct response in internal reality and their finding the actual correct interpretation in external reality.[2] Such transitional relatedness fosters the development of the patient's differentiated object relation to the analyst both in and out of the transference. At the end of the analysis, when patients carry the analytic object away with them, they leave the transitional object of the analyst's interpretations behind.

These observations apply in some measure to all patients, but they are especially germane in considering the developmentally arrested patient. Such an individual is less able to differentiate the analyst from the analyst's interpretations and from the other nonspecific elements of the psychoanalytic setting. For such a patient, the interpretation and the setting *are* the analyst, and both may be experienced as equivalent to aspects of the self.

This observation helps to account for the therapeutic action of the treatment of developmentally arrested patients. For such individuals the capacity to relate to the analyst's correct verbal interventions as transitional objects is a developmental advance that facilitates the development of a capacity for symbolic mental representation. Once these patients can relate to the interpretation as a transitional object, they can *create* the interpretation, *use* it, *find themselves* in it, and eventually *discard* it.[3] Within this developmental line, the response to the incorrect interpretation is as crucial as the response to the correct interpretation. For example, patients frequently react to disappointments in the analytic setting with disturbances of self-experience, and some patients may react with acting out, suicidal despair, or other fragmentation symptoms. Recognizing this, Kohut and Wolf (1978) stated:

---

[2]Recently, Atwood and Stolorow (1984) and Ogden (1994), in particular, have expanded on the notion of the intersubjective aspects of the psychoanalytic encounter.

[3]In unduly prolonged analyses, interpretations may have been pathologically transformed by the patient and analyst from transitional objects into fetish objects that cannot be relinquished (D. Rinsley, personal communication, January 1986).

If a normally tastefully dressed patient arrives in our office in a disheveled attire, if his tie is grossly mismatched, and the colour of his socks does not go with that of his shoes, we shall usually not go wrong if we begin to search our memory with the question whether we had been unempathic in the last session, whether we had failed to recognize a narcissistic need. (p. 418)

Winnicott (1971b), writing about the infant's experience of mirroring, described an infant nursing at the breast. Ordinarily, the infant is not looking at the breast but into the mother's face. Winnicott wrote "What does the baby see when he or she looks at the mother's face? I am suggesting that, ordinarily, what the baby sees is himself or herself. In other words, the mother is looking at the baby and *what she looks like is related to what she sees there*" (p. 112; emphasis in original).

Winnicott pointed the way to a fuller understanding of how the self-representation is internalized through a scanning of the mother. The reciprocal of this is that *the mother in some sense also looks like how the infant feels,* so that the object representation becomes objectified by an externalization of the self-representation (Kumin, 1986). The mutual interchange between self- and object representations, inside and outside, lays the foundation for the infant's later capacity to find a transitional object as well as for the much later ability to form a transitional relationship to the correct intervention or the correct verbal interpretation.

In contrast is the situation Winnicott described a few paragraphs later: "A baby so treated [to maternal failure in the realm of empathic handling] will grow up puzzled about mirrors and what the mirror has to offer. If the mother's face is unresponsive, then a mirror is a thing to be looked at but not to be looked into" (p. 113). In the same way that the relation to the mother's face is not yet wholly differentiated from the self-representation, developmentally arrested patients find it difficult to look into themselves in the mirror of the analyst's interpretations. Just as a "false self" (Winnicott, 1960b) hides and protects the core identity from invasion and trauma, so too are resistance and collusive compliance the patient's self-protective transference relations to the incorrect interpretation, imagined or real.

The infant's "puzzlement" about mirrors, its incapacity to look into them, is a precocious defense. To the extent that the infant has had to organize defenses against failures of maternal empathy, it will have an impaired capacity in the realm of transitional relating. Instead of a transitional object the infant must form a defensively premature object relationship to what is absent. At such an early stage of development, the distinction between a primitive identification and an object relation is not yet formed. Therefore, infants experience something missing in themselves, and in some sense it *is* missing. The patient did look into the mirror of the mother's face and does look into the mirror of the analyst's interpretation but sees nothing of himself or herself; all that is seen is the mirror's frame, signifying the outline of an object's presence, although the object is transparent and contains no link to or reflection of the self. The pre-object deprivation in the experience of the mother and the analyst leads to an inner sense of emptiness.[4] If the interpretation or attunement (Eigen, 1973) is incorrect, the patient may appear withdrawn from the analyst and hypo- or hyperactive because, from the patient's point of view, the analyst is evanescent. The patient sees nothing of himself or herself because the analyst has seen nothing.

If part of the patient's self-representation is repeatedly seen as nothing, it eventually becomes evacuated and empty. What is missing from the self-representation is cathected, but it is cathected negatively (Green, 1975, 1978). According to Green, such patients feel that "all they have is what they have not got." Thus, the correct interpretation, like accurate empathic mirroring, fills and illuminates the transitional space while the incorrect interpretation invades it with its absence, emptying it and making it collapse. The incorrect interpretation replaces a good-enough transitional relationship with pathological pre-object relatedness leading to withdrawn avoidant or ambivalent behavior.

This understanding adds to that of my previous paper on the experience of emptiness (Kumin, 1978a). In that paper I described the structurally deficient ego core[5] of schizoid patients and reported

---

[4]I originally wrote (Kumin, 1989) that "the mother and the analyst are experienced as *empty objects*," although I now understand this disturbance to affect *pre*-object relatedness no less than more subjectively differentiated experiences of object relatedness.

[5]Nowadays I would tend to describe such conditions in the more experience-near terms of a self-representation which is felt to be empty or in the behavioral term of withdrawn relatedness rather than in the experience-distant terms of an ego which is structurally and libidinally hollow (Stolorow, 1978; Stolorow and Atwood, 1979).

the following dream of a schizoid patient in the first weeks of treatment, a dream that I felt typified this experience of inner emptiness:

> *She was alone in an empty house. There was a succession of large rooms, all open and empty, with high ceilings and no furniture. She came to one room which was locked, and to which she could not gain entry. She walked up a stairway which divided. On the top landing was a large mirror. When she looked into it, she saw no one, no reflexion of herself.* (p. 207)

At the time, I primarily saw this dream as typifying the patient's vacant self-representation. But this view would now seem incomplete to me since it does not sufficiently take into account the effect of the patient's pre-object relationships on her self-experience. I had not understood the significance of the *emptiness* of the house in which the dream transpired, the *locked room,* and the containing *frame* of the mirror that *did not reflect her image.* I would now be more likely to speculate that the patient may have been communicating her fear of being retraumatized by me in her psychotherapy. She was fearful that I, like her mother, would not provide for her emotional needs; would bar entry to her communications; and would leave her feeling empty, estranged, and devoid of an adequate representational capacity regarding her self and her affects.

THERAPEUTIC CONSIDERATIONS

In practice, the recognition and analysis of negative reactions to incorrect interpretations prove as helpful as anything else in furthering the patient's treatment and elucidating the nature of the transference. However, it is the timely, accurate, and successful working through of the effects of the previous faulty intervention that is therapeutic. Given a secure therapeutic framework, what moves the analysis forward is ultimately the correct interpretation. In general, four distinct phases can be isolated in this process:

1. Recognition of the patient's perception of an incorrect interpretation
2. Acknowledgment of the analyst's error (either explicitly or implicitly)

3. Rectification of the error by substitution of what would have been the correct interpretation
4. Analysis of the patient's response to the incorrect interpretation

There are times, usually well into an analysis, when the exploration of the patient's response to the analyst's interpretive error leads to a fifth phase, a reconstruction of the origin of the patient's infantile trauma.

At first, analysts must help patients with recognition of all of this emotional truth and falsehood. After a while—sometimes a long while—the patients can do most of this on their own. Once their defensive idealization of the analyst and denial of personal aggression has begun to fade, they will be better able to sort out their own veridical perceptions of interpretive errors from negative transference responses to correct interpretations. This increasing ability is related to, among other factors, the strengthening of patients' capacity to differentiate "me" from "not-me" and to reestablish a natural perspective to their representational world.

It seems to me, however, that analysts must be able to acknowledge their own error, at the very least, to themselves. This is the "rate-limiting step" without which there can occur no further substitution of a correct interpretation, no exploration of the meaning of the patient's response, no reconstruction of the patient's remote past, no mutative analysis of the transference. This does not mean that analysts should necessarily confess these errors to the patient, express guilt over the matter, or allude to their countertransference. They may only compound their error by further burdening the patient. Instead, with a developmentally more advanced patient analysts matter-of-factly interpret the patient's conflict over the perception of the error, just as they would interpret any other conflict concerning the external world.

The analyst must assist developmentally less advanced patients in tracing the morbid transformation of their self-representation to their recent experiences of failure in the therapeutic setting. Some interpretations may contain tacit or explicit acknowledgment of the validity of the patient's perceptions and experience of the analyst's error. I strongly agree with the recent emphasis by several authors (Schwaber, 1981, 1992; Stolorow et al., 1987) on the importance of attunement to the patient's subjective experience of the analyst's failures. The prototype of this view was presented in 1955 by Edward Glover:

> The smallest detail of the analytical setting is as important to the patient as the smallest detail of a dream is to the analyst. The patient reacts, in some cases manifestly, as if it were a *symbol of a danger situation*. Indeed, we cannot realize too soon that all patients, whether they are aware of it or not, interpret the minutiae of analytical life with greater and more consistent skill than does the analyst himself. (p. 26; emphasis in original)

But I would go further and take into account the objective reality of the analyst's failures as potential repetitions in the transference of "actual failures of ego-support that held up the individual's emotional development" (Winnicott, 1963b, p. 207). The analyst must take into account the patient's psychic reality as well as his or her developmental reality (Schafer, 1985) as reproduced in the analytic interaction. The incorrect interpretation is not merely symbolic of a danger situation, it is an *actual* danger situation that both signals and repeats similar danger situations from the past. Winnicott (1963b) addressed this issue as follows:

> In this work the failures of the therapist . . . will be real and they can be shown to reproduce the original failures, in token form. These failures are real indeed, and especially so in so far as the patient is either regressed to the dependence of the appropriate age, or else remembering. The acknowledgment of the analyst's . . . failure enables the patient to become appropriately angry instead of traumatized. (p. 209)

Greenacre (1971) addressed the same issue:

> As I look over cases of patients who have definite disturbances beginning in infancy, I think the understanding of what has happened is probably only effective therapeutically if the analyst has been able to maintain a resilient interest and concern for the patient in the setting of the basic transference situation. The patient has to feel assured of the analyst's concern and his fidelity to their mutual work. This is probably of major importance throughout, much greater than the precision of the interpretation. For this reason I rarely insist on the interpretation even when I think it is substantially correct, though it may not have been timed quite accurately. On the other hand, I think

that with such patients it is difficult to judge the proper timing. Often it is better simply to wait until the situation is again ripe and a revised repetition of the interpretation may then begin to take hold. I am not sure I know why the quality of the basic transference relationship is so important. I have thought that it is largely due to the fact that the analyst serves as a reliable "good enough parent" (to use Winnicott's phrase). This may be a new experience to the patient who is used to finding ambivalence because he himself provokes it. Further, I may feel that I have made a mistake or misunderstood something. I try not to let it slip by, but to admit it clearly. This often is reassuring to the patient who has been used to false reassurances and inaccurate criticisms. (pp. 45–46)

Thus, some occasions may demand explicit acknowledgment, although this is ideally done within the transference and preparatory to the formulation of a reconstruction of the historical roots of the therapeutic interaction. Two examples follow:

Recall the woman I described in Chapter Seven whose past pharmacological treatment for her profound depression had been ineffective and who sought intensive psychotherapy with me. Her psychic state was much like that of the sufferers from severe trauma who were described by Krystal (1978), as having severe psychic numbing, a feeling of emotional "deadness," constriction and blocking of mental processes, dissociation from the past, and a "catatonoid" state verging on lethal psychological surrender. Hardly a day went by when my patient did not seriously consider suicide. In the first year of treatment she responded poorly to my interpretations, frequently feeling even more depleted and suicidal after I made what I felt at the time were accurate interventions that I had intended to be helpful. At times the patient became virtually mute for weeks on end in her sessions.

There were times when I felt close to despair and exhaustion myself, in that my efforts to help the patient only seemed to make matters worse for her. Gradually I began to realize that for the patient psychotherapy itself was a cumulative trauma indistinguishable from her childhood and that my feelings were likely to be similar to those of the patient herself and the internal objects with whom she was identified (especially her mother). What seemed to be germane to an adequate response to the needs of this particular patient was an understanding along the lines of Goldberg's (1979) paper, "Remarks on Transference–Countertransference in Psychotic States." Goldberg, sensitively pointing out that since the earliest experiences of the infant are with the mother's body, the most primitive forms of transference are with the analyst's body, wrote, "While the neurotic transference is directed mainly *onto* the therapist and is handled within the therapist's mind, the psychotic transference, regardless of diagnosis, is directed *into* the therapist's body, and the therapist then experiences it within herself. This requires an additional step in understanding the therapist's role and function and the ultimate meaning of the interpretation—both in its function and in its effect on patient and therapist" (p. 347; emphasis in original).

When the patient now felt more hopeless and suicidal, I was likely to call her attention to the source of her anguish in some actual event, frequently an error of mine. The errors were easy to make, as she provided meager information about the state of her thoughts and feelings. Nevertheless, they were real errors, and they produced real effects on the patient. She initially did not want to think that my lack of understanding could have such a significant effect on her, but she gradually provided ample confirmation of this conjecture. Gradually, the patient and I ceased denying to ourselves that I was failing her and shifted our attention to *how* she felt I was failing her.

One day the patient expressed the feeling that she couldn't talk about her depression to others without them preempting her feelings by telling her that they were also depressed. After the patient and I linked this feeling to numerous recent events relating to others as well as to me, I said I believed that the feeling must also date from an earlier time in her life.

The patient then recalled being told that for an extended time during her infancy her mother had been despondent. At the next session she reported having asked her mother for more information on this time in her life. Her mother told her that when she was six months old her grandmother (the mother of the patient's mother) became severely depressed and came to live with them. During this time the patient's grandmother received a course of outpatient shock therapy and her mother, a nurse, cared for the woman at home. The patient's mother was effectively lost to her suddenly. Moreover, while she nursed the patient's grandmother for an extended period of time she became depressed herself.

Thus, the patient had identified with her emotionally exhausted mother and silently withdrawn grandmother and had internalized these depleted, empty pre-objects as part of her own developing self-representation.

The effect of my acknowledgments that I, like the patient's mother and grandmother, was unwittingly contributing to her depression was to point to a breakdown that at one time in the past was external but was experienced as a part of herself (Green, 1980). Now she could differentiate herself better from the despair of the past situation, react to it, and adapt herself more effectively to it. From this point on the patient's treatment carried a different tone and a markedly diminished sense of hopelessness.

A vignette from Winnicott's *Playing and Reality* (1971b), although a highly idiosyncratic one, may prove even more illuminating about the link between admissions within the transference of therapeutic lapses and subsequent therapeutic reconstructions. Winnicott described the analysis of a middle-aged married man who had a family and success in his profession. Despite much good therapeutic work by Winnicott, previous therapists, and the patient himself, there was still a feeling in this patient that "what he came for he had not reached."

On a Friday the patient came and reported much as usual. The thing that struck me on the Friday was that the patient was talking about *penis envy* . . . .

The change that belongs to this particular phase is shown in the way I handled this. On this particular occasion I said to him: "I am listening to a girl. I know perfectly well that you are a man but I am listening to a girl, and I am talking to a girl. I am telling this girl: 'You are talking about penis envy.' "

It was clear to me, by the profound effect of this interpretation, that my remark was in some way apposite, and indeed I would not be reporting this incident in this context were it not for the fact that the work that started on this Friday did in fact break into a vicious circle. I had grown accustomed to a routine of good work, good interpretations, good immediate results, and then destruction and disillusionment that followed each time because of the patient's gradual recognition that something fundamental had remained unchanged; there was this unknown factor which had kept this man working at his own analysis for a quarter of a century. . . .

On this occasion there was an immediate effect in the form of intellectual acceptance, and relief, and then there were more remote effects. After a pause the patient said: "If I were to tell someone about this girl I would be called mad."

The matter could have been left there, but I am glad, in view of subsequent events, that I went further. It was my next remark that surprised me, and it clinched the matter. I said: "It was not that *you* told this to anyone; it is *I* who see the girl and hear a girl talking, when actually there is a man on my couch. The mad person is *myself*."

I did not have to elaborate this point because it went home. The patient said that he now felt sane in a mad environment. In other words he was now released from a dilemma. . . .

This [acknowledgment of the] madness which was mine enabled him to see himself as a girl *from my position*. He knows himself to be a man, and never doubts that he is a man. . . .

This complex state of affairs has a special reality for this man because he and I have been driven to the conclusion (though unable to prove it) that his mother (who is not alive now) saw a girl baby when she saw him as a baby before she came round to thinking of him as a boy. In other words this man had to fit into her idea that her baby would be and was a girl. (He was the second child, the first being a boy.) We have very good evidence from inside the analysis that in her early management of him the mother held him and dealt with him in all sorts of physical ways as if she failed to see him as a male. On the basis of this pattern he later arranged his defenses, but it was the mother's "madness" that saw a girl where there was a boy, and this was brought right into the present by my having said, "It is I who am mad."

In the subsequent weeks there was a great deal of material confirming the validity of my interpretation and my attitude, and the patient felt that he could see now that his analysis had ceased to be under doom of interminability. (pp. 73–75; emphasis in original)

In this remarkable vignette Winnicott's correct interpretation partly consisted of his acknowledgment to the patient, within the transference, of the reality of two errors he had made. First, he explicitly admitted the madness of hearing a girl talking when the patient was in fact a male. Additionally, Winnicott tacitly assumed responsibility for having failed to recognize the deepest source of the patient's suffering until just then. Every interpretation, even a correct one, simultaneously reveals both the extent as well as the limits of what the analyst has understood. Winnicott dealt with the patient's transference as not solely a fantasied id wish system but simultaneously as a reenacted ego need. In the example above, he accepted the validity of the patient's experience simply and vividly.

Although paradoxical, it is only after the analyst has acknowledged that the patient's experience is based on the perception of what for him is a *current external* reality that the experience can be allowed to enter the patient's awareness as a *past internal* reality. Only this crucial acknowledgment can lead to a reconstruction of the patient's childhood experience, even of the patient's archaic pre-object trauma, and be mediated mutatively within the transference.

Bibliography

Ainsworth, M. D. S. (1962). The effects of maternal deprivation: A review of findings and controversy in the context of research strategy. In *Deprivation of Maternal Care: A Reassessment of its Effects*. Public Health Papers 14. Geneva: World Health Organization.

Ainsworth, M. D. S. (1967). *Infancy in Uganda: Infant Care and the Growth of Attachment*. Baltimore: Johns Hopkins University Press.

Ainsworth, M. D. S. (1969). Object relations, dependency, and attachment: A theoretical review of the infant–mother relationship. *Child Devel.* 40: 969–1025.

Ainsworth, M. D. S. (1973). The development of infant–mother attachment. In *Review of Child Development Research: Volume 3,* Caldwell, B. M., and Ricciuti, H. N., eds. Chicago: University of Chicago Press.

Ainsworth, M. D. S. (1982). Attachment: Retrospect and prospect. In *The Place of Attachment in Human Behavior,* Parkes, C. M., and Stevenson-Hinde, J., eds. New York: Basic Books.

Ainsworth, M. D. S. (1985). I. Patterns of infant–mother attachment: Antecedents and effects on development. II. Attachments across the life span. *Bull. N.Y. Acad. Med.* 6: 771–812.

Ainsworth, M. D. S., Blehar, M. C., Waters, E., and Wall, S. (1978a). *Patterns of Attachment: A Psychological Study of the Strange Situation*. Hillsdale, NJ: Erlbaum.

Ainsworth, M. D. S., Blehar, M. C., Waters, E., and Wall, S. (1978b). *Patterns of Attachment: Assessed in the Strange Situation and at Home*. Hillsdale, NJ: Erlbaum.

Ainsworth, M. D. S., and Wittig, B. A. (1969). Attachment and exploratory behavior of one-year-olds in a strange situation. In *Determinants of Infant Behaviour: Volume 4,* Foss, B. M., ed. London: Methuen.

Altman, L. L. (1977). Some vicissitudes of love. *J. Amer. Psychoanal. Assn.* 25: 35–54.

Anderson, M. K. (1995). "May I bring my newborn baby to my analytic hour?": One analyst's experience with this request. *Psychoanal. Inq.* 15: 358–368.

Anzieu, D. (1989). *The Skin Ego: A Psychoanalytic Approach to the Self.* New Haven, CT: Yale University Press.

Arlow, J. A. (1986). Discussion of papers by Dr. McDougall and Dr. Glasser: Panel on Identification in the Perversions. *Int. J. Psycho-Anal.* 67: 245–250.

Associated Press. (1992, February 28). You can't fool moms of newborn infants, researchers find. *Seattle Post-Intelligencer,* p. E1.

Atwood, G., and Stolorow, R. (1984). *Structures of Subjectivity: Explorations in Psychoanalytic Phenomenology.* Hillsdale, NJ: Analytic Press.

Bach, S. (1975). Narcissism, continuity and the uncanny. *Int. J. Psycho-Anal.* 56: 77–86.

Bak, R. C. (1973). Being in love and object loss. *Int. J. Psycho-Anal.* 54: 1–8.

Baranger, M., and Baranger, W. (1966). Insight in the analytic situation. In *Psychoanalysis in the Americas,* Litman, R. E., ed. New York: International Universities Press.

Basch, M. F. (1983). Empathic understanding: A review of the concept and some theoretical implications. *J. Amer. Psychoanal. Assn.* 31: 101–126.

Basch, M. F. (1985). Interpretation: Toward a developmental model. In *Progress in Self Psychology: Volume One,* Goldberg, A. I., ed. New York: Guilford Press.

Beard, R. M. (1969). *An Outline of Piaget's Developmental Psychology for Students and Teachers.* New York: New American Library, 1972.

Bender, L. (1935). Emotional problems in children. In *Proceedings of the Second Institute on the Exceptional Child.* Langhorne, PA: The Child Research Clinic of the Woods Schools.

Benedek, T. (1977). Ambivalence, passion, and love. *J. Amer. Psychoanal. Assn.* 25: 53–80.

Bennett, S. L. (1976). Infant–caretaker interactions. In *Infant Psychiatry: A New Synthesis,* Rexford, E. N., Sander, L. W., and Shapiro, T., eds. New Haven, CT: Yale University Press.

Bergman, P. and Escalona, S. (1949). Unusual sensitivities in very young children. *Psychoanal. Study Child* 3/4: 333–352.

Bick, E. (1968). The experience of the skin in early object-relations. *Int. J. Psycho-Anal.* 49: 484–486.

Bion, W. R. (1955). Group dynamics: A re-view. In *New Directions in Psycho-Analysis,* Klein, M., Heimann, P., and Money-Kyrle, R., eds. New York: Basic Books.

Bion, W. R. (1957). Differentiation of the psychotic from the nonpsychotic personalities. In *Second Thoughts: Selected Papers on Psychoanalysis.* New York: Jason Aronson, 1967.

Bion, W. R. (1959). Attacks on linking. In *Second Thoughts: Selected Papers on Psycho-Analysis*. New York: Jason Aronson, 1967.

Bion, W. R. (1962a). A theory of thinking. In *Second Thoughts: Selected Papers on Psycho-Analysis*. New York: Jason Aronson, 1967.

Bion, W. R. (1962b). Learning from experience. In *Seven Servants: Four Works by Wilfred R. Bion*. New York: Jason Aronson, 1977.

Bion, W. R. (1963). *Elements of psycho-analysis*. In *Seven Servants: Four Works by Wilfred Bion*. New York: Jason Aronson, 1977.

Bion, W. R. (1967a). Commentary. In *Second Thoughts: Selected Papers on Psycho-Analysis*. New York: Jason Aronson, 1967.

Bion, W. R. (1967b). *Second Thoughts: Selected Papers on Psychoanalysis*. New York: Jason Aronson.

Bion, W. R. (1967c). Notes on memory and desire. In *Classics in Psychoanalytic Technique*, Langs, R., ed. New York: Jason Aronson, 1981.

Bion, W. R. (1977). On a quotation from Freud. In *Borderline Personality Disorders: The Concept, the Syndrome, the Patient*, Hartocollis, P., ed. New York: International University Press.

Blank, M. (1976). The mother's role in infant development: A review. In *Infant Psychiatry: A New Synthesis*, Rexford, E. N., Sander, L. W., and Shapiro, T., eds. New Haven, CT: Yale University Press.

Blum, H. P. (1973). The concept of erotized transference. *J. Amer. Psychoanal. Assn.* 21: 61–76.

Bollas, C. (1987). *The Shadow of the Object: Psychoanalysis of the Unthought Known*. London: Free Associations Press.

Bollas, C. (1989). *Forces of Destiny: Psychoanalysis and Human Idiom*. New York: Jason Aronson.

Bowlby, J. (1951). *Maternal Care and Mental Health*. Geneva: World Health Organization.

Bowlby, J. (1958). The nature of the child's tie to his mother. *Int. J. Psycho-Anal.* 39: 350–373.

Bowlby, J. (1969). *Attachment and Loss: Volume I. Attachment*. New York: Basic Books.

Bowlby, J. (1973). *Attachment and Loss: Volume II. Separation*. New York: Basic Books.

Bowlby, J. (1980). *Attachment and Loss: Volume III. Loss*. New York: Basic Books.

Bowlby, J. (1989). The role of attachment in personality development and psychopathology. In *The Course of Life: Volume I. Infancy*, Greenspan, S. I., and Pollock, G. H., eds. Madison, CT: International University Press.

Brazelton, T. B. (1969). *Infants and Mothers: Differences in Development*. New York: Delacorte Press.

Brazelton, T. B., and Als, H. (1979). Four early stages in the development of mother–infant interaction. *Psychoanal. Study Child* 34: 349–369.

Brazelton, T. B., and Cramer, B. G. (1990). *The Earliest Relationship: Parents, Infants, and the Drama of Early Attachment.* Reading, MA: Addison-Wesley.

Bronk, W. (1985). *Vectors and Smoothable Curves.* San Francisco: North Point Press.

Brothers, L. (1989). A biological perspective on empathy. *Amer. J. Psychiatry* 146: 10–19.

Broucek, F. (1979). Efficacy in infancy: A review of some experimental studies and their possible implications for clinical theory. *Int. J. Psycho-Anal.* 60: 311–316.

Bucci, W. (1985). Dual coding: A cognitive model for psychoanalytic research. *J. Amer. Psychoanal. Assn.* 33: 571–607.

Calef, V., and Weinshel, E. M. (1981). Some clinical consequences of introjection: Gaslighting. *Psychoanal. Q.* 50: 44–66.

Call, J. D., and Marschak, M. (1976). Styles and games in infancy. In *Infant Psychiatry: A New Synthesis,* Rexford, E. N., Sander, L. W., and Shapiro, T., eds. New Haven, CT: Yale University Press.

Casement, P. (1982). Some pressures on the analyst for physical contact during the reliving of an early trauma. *Int. Rev. Psycho-Anal.* 9: 279–286. [Also in Kohon, G., ed. (1986). *The British School of Psychoanalysis: The Independent Tradition.* New Haven, CT: Yale University Press.]

Chasseguet-Smirgel, J. (1985). *The Ego Ideal: A Psychoanalytic Essay on the Malady of the Ideal,* P. Barrows, trans. New York: Basic Books.

Chasseguet-Smirgel, J. (1988). From the archaic matrix of the Oedipus complex to the fully developed Oedipus complex: Theoretical perspective in relation to clinical experience and technique. *Psychoanal. Q.* 57: 505–527.

Cohen, J., and Kinston, W. (1983). Repression theory: A new look at the cornerstone. *Int. J. Psycho-Anal.* 65: 411–422.

Compton, A. (1985). The concept of identification in the work of Freud, Ferenczi, and Abraham: A review and commentary. *Psychoanal. Q.* 54: 200–233.

de Jonghe, F., Rijnierse, P., and Janssen, R. (1991). Aspects of the analytic relationship. *Int. J. Psycho-Anal.* 72: 693–708.

de Jonghe, F., Rijnierse, P., and Janssen, R. (1992). The role of support in psychoanalysis. *J. Amer. Psychoanal. Assn.* 40: 475–499.

de M'Uzan, M. (1978). If I were dead. *Int. Rev. Psycho-Anal.* 5: 485–490.

Deutsch, H. (1942). Some forms of emotional disturbance and their relation to schizophrenia. In *Neuroses and Character Types.* New York: International Universities Press, 1965.

Dorpat, T. L. (1985). *Denial and Defense in the Therapeutic Situation.* New York: Jason Aronson.

Dorpat, T. L. (1991). The primary process revisited. *Soc. Psychoanal. Psychother. Bull.* 6: 5–22.

Dorpat, T. L., and Miller, M. L. (1992). *Clinical Interaction and the Analysis of Meaning: A New Psychoanalytic Theory.* Hillsdale, NJ: Analytic Press.

Dowling, S. (1982). Dreams and dreaming in relation to trauma in childhood. *Int. J. Psycho-Anal.* 63: 157–166.

Eigen, M. (1973). Abstinence and the schizoid ego. *Int. J. Psycho-Anal.* 54: 493–498.

Emde, R. N. (1983). The prerepresentational self and its affective core. *Psychoanal. Study Child* 38: 165–192.

Emde, R. N. (1984). The affective self: Continuities and transformations from infancy. In *Frontiers of Infant Psychiatry: Volume II,* Call, J. D., Galenson, E., and Tyson, R. L., eds. New York: Basic Books.

Emde, R. N. (1988a). Development terminable and interminable: I. Innate and motivational factors from infancy. *Int. J. Psycho-Anal.* 69: 23–39.

Emde, R. N. (1988b). Development terminable and interminable. II. Recent psychoanalytic theory and therapeutic considerations. *Int. J. Psycho-Anal.* 69: 283–296.

Emde, R. N. (1989). Toward a psychoanalytic theory of affect: I. The organizational model and its propositions. In *The Course of Life: Volume I. Infancy,* Greenspan, S. I., and Pollock, G. H., eds. Madison, CT: International Universities Press.

Emde, R. N., and Buchsbaum, H. K. (1989). Toward a psychoanalytic theory of affect: II. Emotional development and signaling in infancy. In *The Course of Life: Volume I. Infancy.* Greenspan, S. I., and Pollock, G. H., eds. Madison, CT: International Universities Press.

Emde, R. N., Gaensbauer, T. J., and Harmon, R. J. (1976). Emotional expression in infancy: A biobehavioral study. *Psychol. Issues,* Monograph 37.

Engel, G. (1962). *Psychological Development in Health and Disease.* Philadelphia: W. B. Saunders.

Epstein, A. W. (1992). Categorization: A fundamental of unconscious mental activity. *J. Amer. Acad. Psychoanal.* 20: 91–98.

Erikson, E. H. (1950). *Childhood and Society.* New York: Norton, 1963.

Erikson, E. H. (1968). *Identity: Youth and Crisis.* New York: Norton.

Etchegoyen, A. (1993). Latency: A reappraisal. *Int. J. Psycho-Anal.* 74: 347–358.

Fagan, J. (1974). The third-degree impasse and schizophrenia. *Voices* (Summer): 4–6.

Fairbairn, W. R. D. (1944). Endopsychic structure considered in terms of object-relationships. In *Psychoanalytic Studies of the Personality.* London: Routledge & Kegan Paul.

Fairbairn, W. R. D. (1952). *Psychoanalytic Studies of the Personality.* London: Routledge & Kegan Paul.

Fairbairn, W. R. D. (1954). Synopsis of an object-relations theory of the personality. *Int. J. Psycho-Anal.* 35: 224–225.

Fairbairn, W. R. D. (1958). On the nature and aims of the Psycho-Analytical treatment. *Int. J. Psycho-Anal.* 39: 374–385.

Federn, P. (1932). Ego feeling in dreams. In *Ego Psychology and the Psychoses,* Weiss, E., ed. New York: Basic Books, 1952.

Federn, P. (1952). *Ego Psychology and the Psychoses,* Weiss, E., ed. New York: Basic Books.

Fenichel, O. (1945). *The Psychoanalytical Theory of the Neuroses.* New York: Norton.

Fonagy, P., Steele, M., Moran, G., Steele, H., and Higgitt, A. (1993). Measuring the ghost in the nursery: An empirical study of the relation between parents' mental representations of childhood experiences and their infants' security of attachment. *J. Amer. Psychoanal. Assn.* 41: 957–989.

Freud, A. (1936) *The Ego and the Mechanisms of Defense.* New York: International Universities Press, 1966.

Freud, A., with Sandler, J. (1981). Discussions in the Hampstead Index on the ego and the mechanisms of defense: II. The application of analytic technique to the study of the psychic institutions. *Bull. Hampstead Clinic* 4: 5–31.

Freud, S. (1900). The interpretation of dreams. *S.E.* 4, 5.

Freud, S. (1905). Three essays on the theory of sexuality. *S.E.* 7: 135–243.

Freud, S. (1910a). A special type of object choice made by men. *S.E.* 11: 165–175.

Freud, S. (1910b). The antithetical meaning of primal words. *S.E.* 11: 153–161.

Freud, S. (1912). The dynamics of transference. *S.E.* 12: 97–108.

Freud, S. (1913). The theme of the three caskets. *S.E.* 12: 289–301.

Freud, S. (1914a). Remembering, repeating and working through (further recommendations on the technique of Psycho-Analysis II). *S.E.* 12: 147–156.

Freud, S. (1914b). On narcissism. *S.E.* 14: 73–102.

Freud, S. (1914c). Observations on transference-love. *S.E.* 12: 157–168.

Freud, S. (1915a). Instincts and their vicissitudes. *S.E.* 14: 117–140.

Freud, S. (1915b). Repression. *S.E.* 14: 141–158.

Freud, S. (1917a). Mourning and melancholia. *S.E.* 14: 243–258.

Freud, S. (1917b). A metapsychological supplement to the theory of dreams. *S.E.* 14: 222–235.

Freud, S. (1918). From the history of an infantile neurosis. *S.E.* 17: 7–122.

Freud, S. (1920). Beyond the pleasure principle. *S.E.* 18: 7–64.

Freud, S. (1921). Group psychology and the analysis of the ego. *S.E.* 18: 69–143.

Freud, S. (1923). The ego and the id. *S.E.* 19: 1–59.

Freud, S. (1925a). A note upon the mystic writing-pad. *S.E.* 19: 227–234.

Freud, S. (1925b). Some additional notes on dream-interpretation as a whole. *S.E.* 19: 127–138.

Freud, S. (1926). Inhibitions, symptoms and anxiety. *S.E.* 20: 87–172.

Freud, S. (1933). New introductory lectures on Psycho-Analysis. *S.E.* 22: 5–182.

Freud, S. (1940). An outline of psychoanalysis. *S.E.* 23: 144–207.

Furman, R. A. (1987). *A pathological form of projective identification.* Unpublished manuscript.

Furman, R. A., and Furman, E. (1984). Intermittent decathexis: A type of parental dysfunction. *Int. J. Psycho-Anal.* 65: 423–434.

Gaddini, E. (1969). On imitation. *Int. J. Psycho-Anal.* 50: 475–484. [Also In Gaddini, E. (1992). *A Psychoanalytic Theory of Infantile Experience: Conceptual and Clinical Reflections,* Limentani, A., ed. London: Tavistock/Routledge.]

Gaddini, E. (1982). Acting out in the psychoanalytic session. *Int. J. Psycho-Anal.* 63: 57–64. [Also in Gaddini, E. (1992). *A Psychoanalytic Theory of Infantile Experience: Conceptual and Clinical Reflections,* Limentani, A., ed. London: Tavistock/Routledge.]

Gaddini, E. (1992). Therapeutic technique in psychoanalysis: Research, controversies, and evolution. In *A Psychoanalytic Theory of Infantile Experience: Conceptual and Clinical Reflections,* Limentani, A., ed. London: Tavistock/Routledge.

Gaddini, R. (1978). Transitional object origins and the psychosomatic symptom. In *Between Reality and Fantasy: Transitional Objects and Phenomena,* Grolnick, S. A., and Barkin, L., eds., in collaboration with Muensterberger, W. New York: Jason Aronson.

Gass, W. H. (1976). *On Being Blue: A Philosophical Inquiry.* Boston: David R. Godine.

Gedo, J. E. (1979). *Beyond Interpretation.* New York: International Universities Press.

Gedo, J. E. (1991). *The hierarchical model of mental functioning, self-organization, repetition, and apraxia.* Unpublished manuscript.

Gill, M. (1982a). *Analysis of Transference: Volume I. Theory and Technique.* New York: International Universities Press.

Gill, M. (1982a). *Analysis of Transference: Volume II. Studies of Nine Audio-Recorded Psychoanalytic Sessions.* New York: International Universities Press.

Glenn, J. (1978). General principles of child analysis. In *Child Analysis and Therapy,* Glenn, J., ed. New York: Jason Aronson.

Glover, E. (1931). The therapeutic effect of inexact interpretation: A contribution to the theory of suggestion. *Int. J. Psycho-Anal.* 12: 397–411.

Glover, E. (1955). *The Technique of Psychoanalysis.* New York: International Universities Press.

Goldberg, L. (1979). Remarks on transference-countertransference in psychotic states. *Int. J. Psycho-Anal.* 60: 347–356.

Goldfarb, W. (1943). Infant rearing and problem behavior. *Amer. J. Orthopsychiat.* 13: 249–265.

Gould, L. (1991). *Female Perversions.* New York: Anchor Books.

Green, A. (1975). The analyst, symbolization and absence in the analytic setting: On changes in analytic practice and analytic experience. *Int. J. Psycho-Anal.* 56: 1–22.

Green, A. (1978). Potential space in psychoanalysis: The object in the setting. In *Between Reality and Fantasy: Transitional Objects and Phenomena,* Grolnick, S. A., and Barkin, L., eds., in collaboration with Muensterberger, W. New York: Jason Aronson.

Green, A. (1980). The dead mother. In *On Private Madness.* Madison, CT: International Universities Press, 1986.

Green, A. (1981). Projection: From projective identification to project. In *Object and Self: A Developmental Approach. Essays in Honor of Edith Jacobson,* Tuttman, S., Kaye, C., and Zimmerman, M., eds. New York: International Universities Press. [Also in Green, A. (1986). *On Private Madness.* Madison, CT: International Universities Press.]

Greenacre, P. (1952). *Trauma, Growth, and Personality.* New York: Norton.

Greenacre, P. (1971). *Emotional Growth.* New York: International Universities Press.

Greene, W. A., Jr. (1958). The role of a vicarious object in the adaptation to object loss: Use of a vicarious object as a means of adjustment to a separation from a significant person. *Psychosoma. Med.* 20: 124–144.

Greenspan, S. (1981). *Psychopathology and Adaptation in Infancy and Early Childhood.* New York: International Universities Press.

Greenspan, S. (1987). *Infants in Multirisk Families.* Madison, CT: International Universities Press.

Greenspan, S. (1989). *The Development of the Ego.* Madison, CT: International Universities Press.

Greenspan, S. (1992). *Infancy and Early Childhood.* Madison, CT: International Universities Press.

Grinberg, L. (1987). Dreams and acting out. *Psychoanal. Q.* 56: 155–176.

Grinberg, L. and Grinberg, R. (1960). Los sueños del día lunes. *Rev. Psicoanal.* 17: 449–455.

Grotstein, J. S. (1985). *Splitting and Projective Identification.* Northvale, NJ: Jason Aronson.

Grotstein, J. S. (1989). The "black hole" as the basic psychotic experience: Some newer psychoanalytic and neuroscience perspectives on psychosis. *J. Amer. Acad. Psychoanal.*

Grotstein, J. S. (1990). Nothingness, meaninglessness, chaos, and the "black hole." *Contemp. Psychoanal.* 26: 377–407.

Guntrip, H. (1961). *Personality Structure and Human Interaction.* New York: International Universities Press.

Guntrip, H. (1968). *Schizoid Phenomena, Object Relations and the Self.* New York: International Universities Press.

Hamilton, V. (1989). "The mantle of safety": Transference interpretation and reconstruction of childhood traumas in once-weekly therapy with a 37-year-old woman. *Winnicott Stud.* 1: 70–97.

Harlow, H. F., and Zimmerman, R. R. (1959). Affectional responses in the infant monkey. *Science* 130: 421–432.

Hartmann, H. (1948). Comments on the psychoanalytic theory of instinctual drives. In *Essays on Ego Psychology: Selected Problems in Psychoanalytic Theory.* New York: International Universities Press, 1964.

Hartmann, H. (1950a). Psychoanalysis and developmental psychology. In *Essays on Ego Psychology: Selected Problems in Psychoanalytic Theory.* New York: International Universities Press, 1964.

Hartmann, H. (1950b). Comments on the psychoanalytic theory of the ego. In *Essays on Ego Psychology: Selected Problems in Psychoanalytic Theory.* New York: International Universities Press, 1964.

Hartmann, H. (1953). Contribution to the metapsychology of schizophrenia. In *Essays on Ego Psychology: Selected Problems in Psychoanalytic Theory.* New York: International Universities Press, 1964.

Hartmann, H. (1955). On the theory of sublimation. In *Essays on Ego Psychology: Selected Problems in Psychoanalytic Theory.* New York: International Universities Press, 1964.

Hartmann, H. (1964). *Essays on Ego Psychology: Selected Problems in Psychoanalytic Theory.* New York: International Universities Press.

Heath, R. (1964). Pleasure response of human subjects to direct stimulation of the brain. In *The Role of Pleasure in Behavior,* Heath, R., ed. New York: Hoeber/Harper & Row.

Heath, R., and Gallant, D. (1964). Activity of the human brain during emotional thought. In *The Role of Pleasure in Behavior,* Heath, R., ed. New York: Hoeber/Harper & Row.

Heimann, P. (1950). On counter-transference. *Int. J. Psycho-Anal.* 31.

Hinde, R. A., and Spencer-Booth, Y. (1971). Effects of brief separation from mother on rhesus monkeys. *Science* 173: 111–118.

Hoffer, W. (1949). Mouth, hand, and ego-integration. *Psychoanal. Study Child* 3/4: 49–56.

Holt, R. R. (1967). The development of the primary process: A structural view. In *Motives and Thought: Psychoanalytic Essays in Honor of David Rapaport*. Holt, R. R., ed. New York: International Universities Press. [Also in Holt, R. R. *Psychol. Issues,* Monograph 18/19.]

Isakower, O. (1938). A contribution to the patho-psychology of phenomena associated with falling asleep. *Int. J. Psycho-Anal.* 19: 331–345.

Izard, C. E. (1971). *The Face of Emotion.* New York: Meredith and Appleton-Century-Crofts.

Jacobs, T. J. (1983). The analyst and the patient's object world: Notes on an aspect of countertransference. *J. Amer. Psychoanal. Assn.* 31: 619–642.

James, M. (1960). Premature ego development: Some observations on disturbances in the first three months of life. *Int. J. Psycho-Anal.* 41: 288–294. [Also in Kohon, G., ed. (1986). *The British School of Psychoanalysis: The Independent Tradition.* New Haven, CT: Yale University Press.]

James, M. (1972). Preverbal communications. In *Tactics and Techniques in Psychoanalytic Therapy.* Science House.

Joseph, B. (1987). Projective identification: Clinical aspects. In *Projection, Identification, Projective Identification,* Sandler, J., ed. Madison, CT: International Universities Press.

Kelman, H. (1975). The "day precipitate" of dreams: The Morris hypothesis. *Int. J. Psycho-Anal.* 56: 209–218.

Kernberg, O. (1966). Structural derivatives of object relationships. *Int. J. Psycho-Anal.* 47: 236–253.

Kernberg, O. (1970). A psychoanalytic classification of character pathology. *J. Am. Psychoanal. Assn.* 18: 800–822.

Kernberg, O. (1975). *Borderline Conditions and Pathological Narcissism.* New York: Jason Aronson.

Kernberg, O. (1976). *Object Relations Theory and Clinical Psycho-Analysis.* New York: Jason Jason Aronson.

Kernberg, O. (1977). Boundaries and structure in love relations. *J. Amer. Psychoanal. Assn.* 25: 81–114. [Also in Kernberg, O. (1980). *Internal World and External Reality: Object Relations Theory Applied.* New York: Jason Aronson.]

Kernberg, O. (1987). Projection and projective identification: Developmental and clinical aspects. In *Projection, Identification, Projective Identification,* Sandler, J., ed. Madison, CT: International Universities Press.

Khan, M. M. R. (1963). The concept of cumulative trauma. *Psychoanal. Study Child* 18: 286–306.

Khan, M. M. R. (1979a). Role of the "collated internal object" in perversion-formations. In *Alienation in Perversions*. New York: International Universities Press.

Khan, M. M. R. (1979b). *Alienation in Perversions*. New York: International Universities Press.

Khan, M. M. R. (1983). *Hidden Selves: Between Theory and Practice in Psychoanalysis*. New York: International Universities Press.

King, K. R., and Dorpat, T. L. (1990). Daddy's girl: An interactional perspective on the transference of defense in the psychoanalysis of a case of father–daughter incest. In *Psychoanalytic Perspectives on Women*, Siegel, E. V., ed. New York: Brunner/Mazel.

Kinston, W., and Cohen, J. (1986). Primal repression: Clinical and theoretical aspects. *Int. J. Psycho-Anal.* 67: 337–355.

Klein, J. (1989). The vestiges of our early attachments become the rudiments of our later well-being. *Winnicott Stud.* 4: 11–21.

Klein, M. (1935). A contribution to the psychogenesis of manic–depressive states. In *Contributions to Psycho-Analysis*. London: Hogarth Press, 1948.

Klein, M. (1946). Notes on some schizoid mechanisms. In *Developments in Psycho-Analysis*, Klein, M., Heimann, P., Isaacs, S., and Riviere, J., eds. London: Hogarth Press and the Institute for Psycho-Analysis, 1952.

Klein, M. (1955). On identification. In *New Directions in Psycho-Analysis*. Klein, M., Heimann, P., and Money-Kyrle, R., eds. New York: Basic Books.

Klein, M., Heimann, P., Isaacs, S., and Riviere, J. (1952). *Developments in Psycho-Analysis*. London: Hogarth Press.

Klein, S. (1980). Autistic phenomena in neurotic patients. *Int. J. Psycho-Anal.* 61: 395–402.

Kohon, G., ed. (1986). *The British School of Psychoanalysis: The Independent Tradition*. New Haven, CT: Yale University Press.

Kohut, H. (1966). Forms and transformations of narcissism. *J. Amer. Psychoanal. Assn.* 14: 243–272.

Kohut, H. (1971). *The Analysis of the Self: A Systematic Approach to the Psychoanalytic Treatment of Narcissistic Personality Disorders*. New York: International Universities Press.

Kohut, H. (1977). *The Restoration of the Self*. New York: International Universities Press.

Kohut, H., and Wolf, E. S. (1978). The disorders of the self and their treatment: An outline. *Int. J. Psycho-Anal.* 59: 413–425.

Krystal, H. (1978). Trauma and affects. *Psychoanal. Study Child* 33: 81–116.

Krystal, H. (1988). *Integration and Self-Healing: Affect, Trauma, Alexithymia*. Hillsdale, NJ: Analytic Press.

Krystal, H. (1990). An information processing view of object-relations. *Psychoanal. Inq.* 10: 221–251.

Kuhl, P. K., and Meltzoff, A. N. (1982). The bimodal perception of speech in infancy. *Science* 218: 1138–1141.

Kuhl, P. K., and Meltzoff, A. N. (1984). The intermodal representation of speech in infants. *Infant Behav. Devel.* 7: 361–381.

Kumin, I. M. (1978a). Emptiness and its relation to schizoid ego structure. *Int. Rev. Psycho-Anal.* 5: 207–216.

Kumin, I. M. (1978b). Developmental aspects of opposites and paradox. *Int. Rev. Psycho-Anal.* 5: 477–484.

Kumin, I. (1985). *Difficulties in the psychoanalytic concept of the self.* Unpublished manuscript.

Kumin, I. (1985–1986). Erotic horror: Desire and resistance in the psycho-analytic situation. *Int. J. Psychoanal. Psychother.* 11: 3–20.

Kumin, I. (1986). "The shadow of the object": Notes on self- and object-representations. *Psychoanal. Contemp. Thought* 9: 653–675.

Kumin, I. (1989). The incorrect interpretation. *Int. J. Psycho-Anal.* 70: 141–152.

Lacan, J. (1949). The mirror stage as formative of the function of the I as revealed in psychoanalytic experience. In *Ecrits: A Selection,* Sheridan, A., trans. New York: Norton, 1977.

Lacan, J. (1978). *The Four Fundamental Concepts of Psycho-Analysis.* New York: Norton.

Lamb, M. E. (1978). Qualitative aspects of mother– and father–infant attachments. *Infant Behav. Devel.* 1: 165–175.

Lamb, M. E. (1981). Paternal influences on child development: An overview. In *The Role of the Father in Child Development,* Lamb, M. E., ed. New York: Wiley.

Lamb, M. E. (1987). Predictive implications of individual differences in attachment. *J. Consult. Clin. Psychol.* 55: 817–824.

Lamb, M. E., and Easterbrooks, M. A. (1981). Individual differences in parental sensitivity: Origins, components, and consequences. In *Infant Social Cognition: Empirical and Theoretical Considerations,* Lamb, M. E., and Sherrod, L. R., eds. Hillsdale, NJ: Erlbaum.

Langmeier, J., and Matejcek, Z. (1975). *Psychological Deprivation in Childhood.* Queensland, Australia: University of Queensland Press.

Langs, R. (1976). *The Bipersonal Field.* New York: Jason Aronson.

Langs, R. (1977). Some communicative properties of the bipersonal field. In *Technique in Transition.* New York: Jason Aronson.

Langs, R. (1978a). *The Therapeutic Interaction.* New York: Jason Aronson.

Langs, R. (1978b). *Technique in Transition.* New York: Jason Aronson.

Langs, R. (1979). *The Supervisory Experience.* New York: Jason Aronson.

Langs, R. (1980). Truth therapy/lie therapy. In *Classics in Psychoanalytic Technique*. Langs, R., ed. New York: Jason Aronson, 1981.

Langs, R. J., Bucci, W., Udoff, A. L., Cramer, G., and Thomson, L. (1993). Two methods of assessing unconscious communication in psychotherapy. *Psychoanal. Psychol.* 10: 1–16.

Laplanche, J., and Pontalis, J.-B. (1973). *The Language of Psycho-Analysis*. New York: Norton.

Levin, R. (1990). Somatic symptoms, psychoanalytic treatment, emotional growth. In *Psychoanalytic Perspectives on Women*, Siegel, E. V., ed. New York: Brunner/Mazel.

Lewin, B. D. (1946). Sleep, the mouth, and the dream screen. In *Selected Writings of Bertram D. Lewin*, Arlow, J. A., ed. New York: Psychoanalytic Quarterly, 1973.

Lewin, B. D. (1948a). Inferences from the dream screen. In *Selected Writings of Bertram D. Lewin*, Arlow, J. A., ed. New York: Psychoanalytic Quarterly, 1973.

Lewin, B. D. (1948b). The nature of reality, the meaning of nothing, with an addendum on concentration. *Psychoanal Q.* 17: 524–526.

Lipton, S. (1977). Clinical observations on resistance to the transference. *Int. J. Psycho-Anal.* 58: 463–472.

Loewald, H. W. (1960). On the therapeutic action of Psycho-Analysis. *Int. J. Psycho-Anal.* 41: 16–33. [Also in Loewald, H. W. (1980). *Papers on Psychoanalysis*. New Haven, CT: Yale University Press.]

Loewald, H. W. (1973). On internalization. In *Papers on Psychoanalysis*. New Haven, CT: Yale University Press, 1980.

Loewald, H. W. (1980). *Papers on Psychoanalysis*. New Haven, CT: Yale University Press.

Loewald, H. W. (1981). Regression: Some general considerations. *Psychoanal. Q.* 50: 22–43.

Loewald, H. W. (1988). *Sublimation: Inquiries into Theoretical Psychoanalysis*. New Haven, CT: Yale University Press.

Lorenz, R., and Tinbergen, N. (1938). Taxis and instinctive behavior pattern in egg-rolling by the Graylag goose. In *Studies in Animal and in Human Behavior: Volume I*, Lorenz, K., ed., Martin R., trans. Cambridge, MA: Harvard University Press, 1970.

Mahler, M. S. (1968). *On Human Symbiosis and the Vicissitudes of Individuation: Volume 1. Infantile Psychosis*. New York: International Universities Press.

Mahler, M. S., Pine, F., and Bergman, A. (1975). *The Psychological Birth of the Human Infant: Symbiosis and Individuation*. New York: Basic Books.

Main, M. (1977). Analysis of a particular form of reunion behavior seen in some daycare children: Its history and sequelae in children who are home-reared. In *Social Development in Childhood: Daycare Programs and Research*, R. Webb, ed. Baltimore: Johns Hopkins University Press.

Main, M., Kaplan, N., and Cassidy, J. (1985). Security in infancy, childhood and adulthood: A move to the level of representation. In *Growing Points of Attachment Theory and Research: Monographs of the Society for Research in Child Development*, Serial Number 209, Bretherton, I., and Waters, E., eds. Chicago: University Chicago Press.

Main, M., and Stadtman, J. (1981). Infant response to rejection of physical contact by the mother: Aggression, avoidance and conflict. *J. Amer. Acad. Child Psychiat.* 20: 292–307.

Main, M., Tomasini, L., and Tolan, W. (1979). Differences among mothers of infants judged to differ in security. *Developmental Psychol.* 15: 472–473.

Main, M., and Weston, D. R. (1982). Avoidance of the attachment figure in infancy: Descriptions and interpretations. In *The Place of Attachment in Human Behavior*, Parks, C. M., and Stevenson-Hinde, J., eds. New York: Basic Books.

Malin, A., and Grotstein, J. S. (1966). Projective identification in the therapeutic process. *Int. J. Psycho-Anal.* 47: 26–31.

Mangham, C. A. (1981). Insight: Pleasurable affects associated with insight and their origins in infancy. *Psychoanal. Study Child* 36: 271–277.

Manson, B. (1993, December 18). Can mom sleeping with baby reduce SIDS? Study to see. *Seattle Times*, p. 1.

Masterson, J. F., and Rinsley, D. B. (1975). The borderline syndrome: The role of the mother in the genesis and psychic structure of the borderline personality. *Int. J. Psycho-Anal.* 56: 163–177.

McClelland, R. T. (1993). Autistic space. *Psychoanal. Contemp. Thought* 16: 197–231.

Meissner, W. W. (1981). *Internalization in Psychoanalysis*. New York: International Universities Press.

Meltzoff, A. N. (1985). Perception, action, and cognition in early infancy. *Ann. Pediat.* 32: 63–77.

Meltzoff, A. N. (1990). Foundations for developing a concept of self: The role of imitation in relating self to pther and the value of social mirroring, social modeling, and self practice in infancy. In *The Self in Transition: Infancy to Childhood*, Cicchetti, D., and Beeghly, M., eds. Chicago: University of Chicago Press.

Meltzoff, A. N., and Borton, R. (1979). Intermodal matching by human neonates. *Nature* 282: 403–404.

Meltzoff, A. N., and Moore, M. K. (1977). Imitation of facial and manual gestures by human neonates. *Science* 198: 75–78.

Meltzoff, A. N., and Moore, M. K. (1983a). Newborn infants imitate adult facial gestures. *Child Devel.* 54: 72–79.

Meltzoff, A. N., and Moore, M. K. (1983b). The origins of imitation in infancy: Paradigm, phenomena, and theories. In *Advances in Infancy Research, Volume 2*, Lipsitt, L. P., ed. Noorwood, NJ: Ablex.

Meltzoff, A. N., and Moore, M. K. (1992). Early imitation within a functional framework: The importance of person identity, movement, and development. *Infant Behav. Devel.* 15: 479–505.

Modell, A. H. (1984). *Psychoanalysis in a New Context*. Madison, CT: International Universities Press.

Modell, A. H. (1988). The centrality of the psychoanalytic setting and the changing aims of treatment: A perspective from a theory of object relations. *Psychoanal. Q.* 57: 577–596.

Money, J. (1980). The syndrome of abuse dwarfism: Behavioral data and case report. In *Traumatic Abuse and Neglect of Children at Home*, Williams, G., and Money, J., eds. Baltimore: Johns Hopkins University Press.

Needleman, J. (1963). A critical introduction to Ludwig Binswanger's psychoanalysis. In *Being-in-the-World*, Binswanger, L., ed. New York: Basic Books.

The New Columbia Encyclopedia. (1975). New York: Columbia University Press.

Ogden, T. H. (1979). On projective identification. *Int. J. Psycho-Anal.* 60: 357–373.

Ogden, T. H. (1982). *Projective Identification and Psychotherapeutic Technique.* New York: Jason Aronson.

Ogden, T. H. (1986). *The Matrix of the Mind: Object Relations and the Psychoanalytic Dialogue.* Northvale, NJ: Jason Aronson.

Ogden, T. H. (1989a). The concept of the autistic–contiguous position. *Int. J. Psycho-Anal.* 70: 127–140. [Also in Ogden, T. H. (1989b). *The Primitive Edge of Experience.* New York: Jason Aronson.]

Ogden, T. H. (1989b). *The Primitive Edge of Experience.* Northvale, NJ: Jason Aronson.

Ogden, T. H. (1994). *Subjects of Analysis.* Northvale, NJ: Jason Aronson.

Osofsky, J. D. (1987, July 26). *Early Affect Development: Empirical Research.* Panel at the 35th International Psychoanalytical Congress, Montreal.

Osofsky, J. D., and Eberhart-Wright, A. (1988). Affective exchanges between high-risk mothers and infants. *Int. J. Psycho-Anal.* 69: 221–232.

Papousek, M., and Papousek, H. (1979). Early ontogeny of human social interaction: Its biological roots and social dimensions. In *Human Ethology: Claims and Limits of a New Discipline*, von Cranach, M., Foppa, K., Lepenies, W., and Ploog, P., eds. Cambridge: Cambridge University Press.

Paz, O. (1974). *Teatro de Signos/Transparéncias*, Rios, J., ed. Madrid: Espiral/Fundamentos.

Piaget, J. (1950). *Psychology of Intelligence.* Totowa, NJ: Littlefield, Adams.

Piaget, J. (1962). *Play, Dreams, and Imitation in Children,* Gattegno, C., and Hodgson, F. M., trans. New York: Norton. [First published in French 1945.]

Piaget, J., and Inhelder, B. (1969). *The Psychology of the Child,* Weaver, H., trans. New York: Basic Books.

Piaget, J., and Inhelder, B. (1971). *Mental Imagery in the Child.* New York: Basic Books.

Piaget, J., and Inhelder, B. (1973). *Memory and Intelligence.* New York: Basic Books.

Pine, F. (1982). The experience of self: Aspects of its formation, expansion, and vulnerability. *Psychoanal. Study Child* 37: 143–167.

Piontelli, A. (1992). *From Fetus to Child: An Observational and Psychoanalytic Study.* London: Tavistock/Routledge.

Poland, W. S. (1975). Tact as a psychoanalytic function. *Int. J. Psycho-Anal.* 56: 155–162.

Pontalis, J.-B. (1974). Dream as an object. *Int. Rev. Psycho-Anal.* 1: 125–132. [Also in Pontalis, J.-B. (1981). *Frontiers in Psychoanalysis: Between the Dream and Psychic Pain.* New York: International Universities Press.]

Pound, A. (1982). Attachment and maternal depression. In *The Place of Attachment in Human Behavior,* Parks, C. M., and Stevenson-Hinde, J., eds. New York: Basic Books.

Racker, H. (1957). The meanings and uses of countertransference. *Psychoanal. Q.* 26: 303–357.

Racker, H. (1968). *Transference and Countertransference.* New York: International Universities Press.

Raney, J. (1984). *Listening and Interpreting: The Challenge of the Work of Robert Langs.* New York: Jason Aronson.

Ribble, M. (1965). *The Rights of Infants.* New York: Columbia University Press.

Rinsley, D. B. (1982). *Borderline and Other Self Disorders.* New York: Jason Aronson.

Rinsley, D. B. (1985). Notes on the pathogenesis and nosology of borderline and narcissistic personality disorders. *J. Amer. Acad. Psychoanal.* 13: 317–328.

Robertson, J. (1952). *A Two-Year-Old Goes to the Hospital* [Film]. New York: New York University Film Library.

Robertson, J. (1962). Mothering as an influence on early development: A study of well-baby clinic records. *Psychoanal. Study Child* 17: 245–264.

Rosenfeld, H. (1987). *Impasse and Interpretation: Therapeutic and Antitherapeutic Factors in the Psychoanalytic Treatment of Psychotic, Borderline, and Neurotic Patients.* London: Tavistock.

Sagi, A., and Hoffman, M. (1976). Empathic distress in the newborn. *Devel. Psychol.* 12: 175–176.

Sander, L. W. (1983). Polarity, paradox, and the organizing process in development. In *Frontiers of Infant Psychiatry: Volume One,* Call, J. D., Galenson, F., and Tyson, R. L., eds. New York: Basic Books.

Sandler, A.-M. (1977). Beyond eight-month anxiety. *Int. J. Psycho-Anal.* 58: 195–207.

Sandler, J. (1959). On the repetition of early childhood relationships in later psychosomatic disorder. In *The Nature of Stress Disorder.* London: Hutchinson. [Also in Sandler, J., ed. (1987). *From Safety to Superego.* New York: Guilford Press.]

Sandler, J. (1960a). The background of safety. *Int. J. Psycho-Anal.* 41: 352–355.

Sandler, J. (1960b). On the concept of superego. *Psychoanal. Study Child* 15: 128–162.

Sandler, J. (1967). Trauma, strain and development. In *Psychic Trauma,* Furst, S. S., ed. New York: Basic Books.

Sandler, J. (1976). Countertransference and role-responsiveness. *Int. Rev. Psycho-Anal.* 3: 43–47.

Sandler, J. (1987a). The concept of projective identification. In *Projection, Identification, Projective Identification,* Sandler, J., ed. Madison, CT: International Universities Press.

Sandler, J., ed. (1987b). *From Safety to Superego: Selected Papers of Joseph Sandler.* New York: Guilford Press.

Sandler, J., and Rosenblatt, B. (1962). The concept of the representational world. *Psychoanal. Study Child* 17: 128–145.

Sandler, J., and Sandler, A.-M. (1978). On the development of object relationships and affects. *Int. J. Psycho-Anal.* 59: 285–296.

Sarnoff, (1985). *Latency.* New York: Jason Aronson.

Schafer, R. (1968). *Aspects of Internalization.* New York: International Universities Press.

Schafer, R. (1985). Interpretation of psychic reality, developmental influences, and unconscious communication. *J. Amer. Psychoanal. Assn.* 33: 537–554.

Schwaber, E. A. (1981). Empathy: A mode of analytic listening. *Psychoanal. Inq.* 1: 357–392.

Schwaber, E. A. (1992). Countertransference: The analyst's retreat from the patient's vantage point. *Int. J. Psycho-Anal.* 73: 349–362.

Searles, H. F. (1975). The patient as therapist to his analyst. In *Tactics and Techniques in Psychoanalytic Therapy: Volume 2. Countertransference,* Giovacchini, P., ed. New York: Jason Aronson.

Segal, B. M. (in press). The role of pathogenic selfobjects in the development of a form of defensive self. *Psychoanal. Q.*

Settlage, C. F., Bemesderfer, S., Rosenthal, J., Afterman, J., and Spielman, P. M. (1988). *The appeal cycle in early mother–child interaction: The nature and implications of a finding from developmental research.* Unpublished manuscript.

Shapiro, T., and Stern, D. (1989). Psychoanalytic perspectives on the first year of life: The establishment of the ojbect in an effective field. In *The Course of Life: Volume I. Infancy,* Greenspan, S., and Pollock, G., eds. Madison, CT: International Universities Press.

Sharpe, E. F. (1950). *Collected Papers on Psycho-Analysis,* Brierly, M., ed. London: Hogarth.

Sharpe, E. F. (1978). *Dream Analysis.* New York: Brunner/Mazel. [Originally published 1937.]

Shengold, L. (1974). The metaphor of the mirror. *J. Amer. Psychoanal. Assn.* 22: 97–115.

Shengold, L. (1985). Defensive anality and anal narcissism. *Int. J. Psycho-Anal.* 66: 47–73.

Spitz, R. A. (1945). Hospitalism: An enquiry into the genesis of psychiatric conditions in early childhood. *Psychoanal. Study Child* 1: 53–74.

Spitz, R. A. (1946). Anaclitic depression. *Psychoanal. Study Child* 2: 313–342.

Spitz, R. A. (1951). The psychogenic diseases in infancy. *Psychoanal. Study Child* 6: 255–275.

Spitz, R. A. (1965). *The First Year of Life: A Psychoanalytic Study of Normal and Deviant Development of Object Relations.* New York: International Universities Press.

Spitz, R. A. (1959). *A Genetic Field Theory of Ego Formation.* New York: International Universities Press.

Sroufe, L. A. (1985). Attachment classification from the perspective of infant–caregiver relationships and infant temperament. *Child Devel.* 56: 1–14.

Stern, D. N. (1983). The early development of schema of self, other, and "self with other." In *Reflections on Self Psychology,* Lichtenberg, J., and Kaplan, S., eds. Hillsdale, NJ: Analytic Press.

Stern, D. N. (1985a). Affect attunement. In *Frontiers of Infant Psychiatry: Volume 2,* Call, J. D., Galenson, F., and Tyson, R. L., eds. New York: Basic Books.

Stern, D. N. (1985b). *The Interpersonal World of the Infant: A View From Psychoanalysis and Developmental Psychology.* New York: Basic Books.

Stolorow, R. D. (1975). Toward a functional definition of narcissism. *Int. J. Psycho-Anal.* 56: 179–185.

Stolorow, R. D. (1978). The concept of psychic structure: Its metapsychological and clinical psychoanalytic meanings. *Int. Rev. Psycho-Anal.* 5: 313–320.

Stolorow, R. D. (1991). The intersubjective context of intrapsychic experience: A decade of psychoanalytic inquiry. *Psychoanal. Inq.* 11: 171–184.

Stolorow, R. D., and Atwood, G. E. (1979). *Faces in a Cloud: Subjectivity in Personality Theory.* New York: Jason Aronson.

Stolorow, R. D., Brandchaft, B., and Atwood, G. E. (1987). *Psychoanalytic Treatment: An Intersubjective Approach.* Hillsdale, NJ: Analytic Press.

Stone, L. (1961). *The Psychoanalytic Situation.* New York: International Universities Press.

Strachey, J. (1934). The nature of the therapeutic action of psychoanalysis. *Int. J. Psycho-Anal.* 15: 117–126.

Tahka, V. (1987). On the early formation of the mind: I. Differentiation. *Int. J. Psycho-Anal.* 68: 229–250.

Taylor, G. J. (1987). *Psychosomatic Medicine and Contemporary Psychoanalysis.* Madison, CT: International Universities Press.

Taylor, G. J. (1992). Psychoanalysis and psychosomatics: A new synthesis. *J. Amer. Acad. Psychoanal.* 20: 251–275.

Taylor, G. J. (1993). Clinical application of a dysregulation model of illness and disease: A case of spasmodic torticollis. *Int. J. Psycho-Anal.* 74: 581–596.

Tinbergen, N. (1951). *The Study of the Insect.* New York: Oxford University Press.

Tolpin, M. (1971). On the beginnings of a cohesive self. *Psychoanal. Study Child* 26: 316–354.

Tronick, E., Als, H., Adamson, L., Wise, S., and Brazelton, T. B. (1978). The infant's response to entrapment between contradictory messages in face-to-face interaction. *J. Amer. Acad. Child Psychiat.* 17: 1–13.

Tustin, F. (1980). Autistic objects. *Int. Rev. Psycho-Anal.* 7: 27–40.

Tustin, F. (1984). Autistic shapes. *Int. Rev. Psycho-Anal.* 11: 279–290.

Tustin, F. (1986). *Autistic Barriers in Neurotic Patients.* New Haven, CT: Yale University Press.

Tustin, F. (1990). *The Protective Shell in Children and Adults.* London: Karnac.

Tyson, P., and Tyson, R. L. (1990). *Psychoanalytic Theories of Development: An Integration.* New Haven, CT: Yale University Press.

Wallerstein, R. S. (1975). Psychoanalytic perspectives on the problem of reality. In *Psychotherapy and Psychoanalysis.* New York: International Universities Press.

Wallerstein, R. S. (1986). *Forty-Two Lives in Treatment.* New York: Guilford Press.

Wallerstein, R. S. (1990). Psychoanalysis: The common ground. *Int. J. Psycho-Anal.* 71: 3–21.

Wangh, M. (1962). The "evocation of a proxy": A psychological maneuver, its use as a defense, its purposes, and genesis. *Psychoanal. Study Child* 17: 451–469.

Waters, E., and Deane, K. E. (1985). Defining and assessing individual differences in attachment relationships: Q-methodology and the organization of behavior in infancy and early childhood. In *Growing Points of Attachment Theory and Research: Monographs of the Society for Research in Child Development,* Serial Number 209, Bretherton, I., and Waters, E., eds. Chicago: University Chicago Press.

Waters, E., Vaughn, B. E., and Egeland, B. R. (1980). Individual differences in infant–mother attachment relationships at age one: Antecedents in neonatal behavior in an urban, economically disadvantaged sample. *Child Devel.* 51: 208–216.

Weil, J. L. (1992). *Early Deprivation of Empathic Care.* Madison, CT: International Universities Press.

Weiss, J., Sampson, H., and the Mount Zion Psychotherapy Research Group. (1986). *The Psychoanalytic Process.* New York: Guilford Press.

Welles, J., and Wrye, H. K. (1991). The maternal erotic countertransference. *Int. J. Psycho-Anal.* 72: 93–106.

Wexler, M. (1971). Schizophrenia: Conflict and deficiency. *Psychoanal. Q.* 40: 83–99.

Winnicott, D. W. (1947). Hate in the countertransference. In *Collected Papers: Through Paediatrics to Psycho-Analysis.* New York: Basic Books, 1958.

Winnicott, D. W. (1949). The ordinary devoted mother and her baby. In *The Child and the Family.* London: Tavistock, 1957.

Winnicott, D. W. (1954). The depressive position in normal emotional development. In *Collected Papers: Through Paediatrics to Psycho-Analysis.* New York: Basic Books, 1958.

Winnicott, D. W. (1958a). *Collected Papers: Through Paediatrics to Psycho-Analysis.* New York: Basic Books.

Winnicott, D. W. (1958b). The capacity to be alone. *Int. J. Psycho-Anal.* 39: 416–420.

Winnicott, D. W. (1959–1964). Classification: Is there a Psycho-Analytic contribution to psychiatric classification? In *The Maturational Processes and the Facilitating Environment.* New York: International Universities Press, 1965.

Winnicott, D. W. (1960a). Ego distortion in terms of true and false self. In *The Maturational Processes and the Facilitating Environment.* New York: International Universities Press, 1965.

Winnicott, D. W. (1960b). Theory of the parent–infant relationship. In *The Maturational Processes and the Facilitating Environment.* New York: International Universities Press, 1965.

Winnicott, D. W. (1962). Ego integration in child development. In *The*

Maturational Processes and the Facilitating Environment. New York: International Universities Press, 1965.

Winnicott, D. W. (1963a). Communicating and not communicating leading to a study of certain opposites. In *The Maturational Processes and the Facilitating Environment.* New York: International Universities Press, 1965.

Winnicott, D. W. (1963b). Psychotherapy of character disorders. In *The Maturational Processes and the Facilitating Environment.* New York: International Universities Press, 1965.

Winnicott, D. W. (1965). *The Maturational Processes and the Facilitating Environment.* New York: International Universities Press.

Winnicott, D. W. (1967a). Personal communication to R. Gaddini. Cited in Gaddini, R. (1978). Transitional object origins and the psychosomatic symptom. In *Between Reality and Fantasy: Transitional Objects and Phenomena,* Grolnick, S. A., and Barkin L., eds., in collaboration with Muensterberger, W. New York: Jason Aronson.

Winnicott, D. W. (1967b). Mirror-role of mother and family in child development. In *Playing and Reality.* New York: Basic Books, 1971.

Winnicott, D. W. (1971a). On "the use of an object." In *Psycho-Analytic Explorations,* Winnicott, C., Shepherd, R., and Davis, M., eds. Cambridge, MA: Harvard University Press, 1989.

Winnicott, D. W. (1971b). *Playing and Reality.* New York: Basic Books.

Winnicott, D. W. (1974). Fear of breakdown. *Int. Rev. Psycho-Anal.* 1: 103–105. [Also in Winnicott, D. W. (1989). *Psychoanalytic Explorations.* Winnicott, C., Shepherd, R., and Davis, M., eds. Cambridge, MA: Harvard University Press.]

Winnicott, D. W. (1989). *Psycho-Analytic Explorations,* Winnicott, C., Shepherd, R., and Davis, M., eds. Cambridge, MA: Harvard University Press.

Wrye, H. K., and Welles, J. (1989). The maternal erotic transference. *Int. J. Psycho-Anal.* 70: 673–684.

Wrye, H. K., and Welles, J. (1994). *The Narration of Desire: Erotic Transferences and Countertransferences.* Hillsdale, NJ: Analytic Press.

Zetzel, E. R. (1966). The analytic situation. In *Psychoanalysis in the Americas,* Litman, R. E., ed. New York: International Universities Press.

Index